A Fertile Path

A Fertile Path

Guiding the Journey with Mindfulness and Compassion

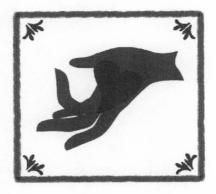

JANETTI MAROTTA, PH.D.

In Partnership with ARC Fertility arc
Foreword by David Adamson, M.D.

This book is intended to be a psycho-educational guide to help reduce the stress of infertility and its treatment. It is not proposed to be a substitute for counseling if needed or for medical assistance or advice. Recommended practices and approaches are generic and may need to be adapted to your individual medical or psychological needs. The author assumes no responsibility for any medical outcomes that may occur as a result of applying the methods suggested in this book. All efforts have been made to assure the accuracy of information at the time of the book's publication.

Cover illustration by Lee Ann O'Neal, LMFT
Chapter head illustrations by Cheyenne Woodward

ISBN: 1975859154
ISBN 13: 9781975859152
Library of Congress Control Number: 2017913410
CreateSpace Independent Publishing Platform
North Charleston, South Carolina

Endorsements

*D*ear reader, you are holding in your hands a treasure trove of wisdom and compassion that can help you with the extraordinary challenges of infertility. A resource like this on your ongoing journey is as precious as a life boat when your ship has struck a reef and can only be offered from the heart of a woman who personally knows the grief and despair of infertility and multiple miscarriages. If you or someone you love has been obliged to bear these burdens, you also know what enormous strength and courage it takes to try again and again.

Janetti Marotta is someone who has traveled and learned to navigate well in these perilous waters, and through the years of her labors, she has gained many precious mindfulness skills like loving kindness and self-compassion as well as emotional self-regulation and resilience. She offers these treasures here to you in abundance. Many blessings for this gift of love and compassion to all who find themselves on this difficult journey. Bon Voyage!

—Steve Flowers, MS, MFT, author of *The Mindful Path through Shyness* and coauthor of *Living with Your Heart Wide Open*

Infertility is a difficult journey and Dr. Marotta demonstrates a way to navigate through the associated stress and uncertainty. Infertility can cause an emotional reaction on par with any other serious life event such as a cancer diagnosis or loss of a loved one. Mindfulness can empower one to deal with all of life's untoward events. You will derive strength and power through this book. Not only will it help throughout the infertility process, the techniques taught in this book will transcend infertility to help with all aspects of life. Mindfulness is more than a powerful support process; it is a way to improve your life. Dr. Marotta has both a compassionate, professional approach and the experience of someone who has gone through the infertility journey. She provides a unique and powerful perspective. I intend to recommend this book as a must read for any couple considering fertility treatment.

> —Hugh S. Taylor, MD, Anita O'Keeffe Young professor and chair in the Department of Obstetrics, Gynecology and Reproductive Sciences, Yale School of Medicine

A Fertile Path is a very wise and compassionate book. It is a loving guide for those living with the not-knowing of fertility. I love how Janetti points again and again to healing—that whether one conceives or not, healing is possible. This is a very important book for those traveling on the journey of fertility and of life itself.

> —Bob Stahl, PhD, coauthor of *A Mindfulness-Based Stress Reduction Workbook, Living with Your Heart Wide Open, Calming the Rush of Panic, A Mindfulness-Based Stress Reduction Workbook for Anxiety, and MBSR Everyday*

Dr. Janetti Marotta puts forth an essential truth; you are most successful in any benevolent venture when you let go, open to what lies before you, and stay connected to the oneness of your mind and body. The path upon which to walk is detailed, engaging, uplifting, and sound—offering every available means to encounter the challenges of your fertility journey.

> —Gregory Sims, PhD, author of *Treating Spiritual Disorders*, coauthor of *Personal Peacefulness*, and cofounder of the American Psychological Association (APA) Division of Peace Psychology

With such compassion and wisdom, Dr. Janetti Marotta offers in *A Fertile Path* an accessible set of holistic practices to cultivate deep resilience and mindful self-care to support you in all aspects of what *your* fertile path may bring you. It is clear that Dr. Marotta has intimately navigated her own fertility journey as her words tenderly capture not only the breadth and depth of the confusion, vulnerability, grief, and stress that this passage may contain but also the potential for deep surrender, healing, and transformation. Reading this vital book is like having a wise, loving friend and mentor walking with you, holding your hand as you find your way.

—Deborah Zucker, ND, author of *The Vitality Map*

A Fertile Path is a beautiful, holistic guide to help you effectively, sanely, and sensitively navigate the complex social and psychological stressors that surround infertility issues and fertility treatments. This is more than a guidebook: the wisdom that fills these pages serves as a supportive friend to accompany you on this life-producing journey. You will find not only profound guidance for creating the most conducive conditions for fertility but life lessons that go far beyond these specific issues and help you create the joyful, mindful, and awake life to which we all so deeply aspire.

—Shaila Catherine, author of *Focused and Fearless: A Meditator's Guide to States of Deep Joy, Calm, and Clarity*

This book is a must read for any woman embarking on, or in the midst of, her fertility journey. It is such an insightful and important combination of supportive actions and information in navigating the Western approach to IVF. This book will help you optimize your fertility potential through mindfulness-based living, as well as help you to broaden your perspective of different family-building options.

—Robin Sheared, LAc, FABORM, clinical director and cofounder of Blue Ova Health

Dr. Marotta has written an uplifting and practical guide for women and men who are experiencing the stress of infertility. Her words are calming and positive. She provides specific suggestions for applying the principles of mindfulness to the fertility journey. I highly recommend this book to anyone experiencing the challenge of infertility.

—Valerie Baker, MD, professor in the Division of Reproductive Endocrinology and Infertility, Stanford University School of Medicine

The journey through the maze of infertility treatments can at times be quite overwhelming. In *A Fertile Path*, Dr. Marotta will provide any reader a blueprint of coping methods and practices that can help make an inevitably stressful journey more tolerable and ultimately more successful. The emphasis on a holistic, compassionate approach, frequently overlooked by patients and providers alike, underscores the importance of the mind-body connection. The methods addressed in this book may also be applied to many other stressful, challenging aspects of life. Whether you are struggling to overcome infertility, or dealing with any other stress inducing obstacles, I recommend the approaches outlined in this book.

—Joel Batzofin, MD, FACOG, medical director of New York Fertility Services and author of *One Step at a Time*

Here's what group participants of the program have to say!

If you're struggling with infertility, this program is invaluable! It will help you restore yourself, your heart, and your outlook and give you strength and tools to continue on this heartbreaking journey. It was worth every single penny, and in a way, it saved my life!

This program helped me find the value of myself again. I learned and accepted that I am more than my fertility treatments…

The Mind-Body Program with Janetti has been extremely helpful to me in maintaining my sanity throughout this fertility journey. She has helped me to look at this process in a different, more positive way. Coming to the place of needing fertility treatments was never something I planned or wanted to do. Participating in the program has helped me come to peace with my decisions for treatment and the possibilities of having non-genetic children. It is a challenging journey, but I have come to see the benefits and growth opportunities that are inherent to the process. I'm a different person than I was at the beginning. I had no idea I could be so poised and comfortable while going through an IVF cycle that was always at the risk of being cancelled. Highly recommended!

I used to think that I handled stress well. This experience with infertility opened my eyes to the reality that this was not so. The program is a gift, a blessing that eased my path in a way I had not expected, nor hoped to expect...

To my daughter Cheyenne, who taught me every child,
however he or she finds a way home to you,
is a child of the universe
and a gift from beyond.

With all my heart.

Contents

Endorsements ·v

Foreword ·xvii

Preface · xix

Acknowledgments · xxiii

Introduction ·xxv

One   **Turning on the Relaxation Response** · · · · · · · · · · · · · · · · 1

       The Paradox of Infertility · 1

       The Paradox of Mindfulness · 4

       Taking the First Step · 6

       Stress, Fertility, and the Mind-Body Connection · · · · · · · 7

       Exercise: Infertility Stress Test · · · · · · · · · · · · · · · · · 9

       The Relaxation Response ·10

       Exercise: Belly Breathing ·11

       Staying the Course of Treatment · · · · · · · · · · · · · · · · ·13

       Breath-Awareness Meditation · · · · · · · · · · · · · · · · · ·14

       Formal Practice: Breath-Awareness Meditation · · · · · · · ·14

       Informal Practice: Belly-Breathing Awareness—Felt · · · · ·15

Two   **Anchoring to the Breath** ·19

       Nowhere Is Now Here · 20

       Mindfulness, MBSR, and Meditation · · · · · · · · · · · · · · 22

       The Formal Practice ·23

       Meditation on the Breath · 28

       Formal Practice: Meditation on the Breath · · · · · · · · · · · 28

	The Informal Practice · 30
	Informal Practice: Breath Awareness—Pause · · · · · · · · · 30
	Navigating Treatment ·31
	Journal: Overall Bank Account · · · · · · · · · · · · · · · · · · 34
	Exercise: Visualization ·35
	Exercise: Map ·37
	Mindful Inquiry: Obstacle Versus Challenge · · · · · · · · · ·38
Three	**Befriending the Body** ·41
	Steering toward Discomfort · 42
	Meditation on the Body · 42
	Formal Practice: Meditation on the Body · · · · · · · · · · · 43
	Informal Practice: Body Awareness—Pause· · · · · · · · · · 44
	Finding Your Edge through Yoga · · · · · · · · · · · · · · · · ·45
	Mindful Yoga for Fertility · 46
	Formal Practice: Mindful Yoga For Fertility · · · · · · · · · 48
Four	**Rejuvenating Holistically** ·56
	Journey, Not Destination ·57
	Boosting Fertility ·58
	Exercise: Fertile Lifestyle Plan · · · · · · · · · · · · · · · · · · ·65
	Mindful Eating· ·67
	Informal Practice: Mindful Eating · · · · · · · · · · · · · · · ·69
	Walking Meditation ·70
	Formal Practice: Walking Meditation · · · · · · · · · · · · · ·71
Five	**Working with Thoughts Skillfully** · · · · · · · · · · · · · · · · · ·76
	Breaking Free by Turning Toward· · · · · · · · · · · · · · · · · 77
	From Looking to Seeing · 80
	Exercise: Power of Thoughts ·81
	Reframing the Journey ·82
	Exercise: Inviting Wholesome Thoughts to Arise · · · · · · 84
	Exercise: Reframe Reminders · · · · · · · · · · · · · · · · · · · 84
	Exercise: Visualization to Work with Thoughts· · · · · · · · 86
	Choiceless Awareness· ·87
	Formal Practice: Choiceless Awareness · · · · · · · · · · · · · ·88

Meditation on Thoughts ·89
Formal Practice: Meditation on Thoughts· · · · · · · · · · · · 90
Informal Practice: Cognitive Awareness · · · · · · · · · · · · ·91

Six   **Making Space for Emotions** · 94
Welcoming the Unwelcome· ·95
Meditation on Emotions · 97
Formal Meditation: Meditation on Emotions · · · · · · · · · ·98
Informal Practice: Emotional Awareness· · · · · · · · · · · · 99
The Grieving Process · 99

Seven   **Meeting Challenging Situations**· · · · · · · · · · · · · · · · · · · ·107
Being the Change Itself· ·108
The Comparing Mind· ·108
Meeting Trying Comments· 110
Encountering Difficult Circumstances · · · · · · · · · · · · · · 114
Journal: Challenging Situations· · · · · · · · · · · · · · · · · · · 116
Intentions of Well-Being · 116
Exercise: Seeds of Intention · 118
Loving-Kindness· 118
Formal Meditation: Loving-Kindness Meditation · · · · · · 119
Informal Practice: Cultivating Loving-Kindness · · · · · · · 121

Eight   **Finding Balance in Relationships**· · · · · · · · · · · · · · · · · · · ·124
Crisis as Opportunity ·125
Understanding Differences ·125
Where Yin Meets Yang · 132
Wise Speech ·133
Exercise: Paired Listening ·134
Exercise: Active Listening ·135
Informal Practice: Cultivating Wise Speech · · · · · · · · · ·136
Chi Kung ·136
Formal Practice: Chi Kung ·137

Nine   **Opening to Family-Building Options** · · · · · · · · · · · · · ·142
Loving the Questions ·143
The World of Adoption· ·144

The Possibilities of Gamete Donation · · · · · · · · · · · · · ·148
The Heart of Surrogacy· ·154
Disclosing Birth Rite· ·157
Exercise: Active Listening ·159
Smiling with Gratitude ·160
Exercise: What's Not Wrong—The Gratitude List · · · · ·161
Informal Practice: Cultivating Gratitude· · · · · · · · · · · ·162
Aspiration Meditation· ·162
Formal Practice: Aspiration Meditation· · · · · · · · · · · · ·162
Mindful Inquiry: Pregnancy Versus Parenthood · · · · · ·163

Ten   **Giving Birth to Yourself** ·166
Nothing Is Everything ·167
Informal Practice: Cultivating Generosity· · · · · · · · · · ·167
Tonglen· ·167
Formal Practice: Tonglen ·168
Returning to Your Deep Intention · · · · · · · · · · · · · · ·169

Epilogue· ·173
Appendix Fertility 101 ·177
Resources· ·185
References ·189
About the Author· ·197

Foreword

*I*n the last two decades, assisted reproductive technology (ART) has afforded the opportunity for thousands to close the gap between infertility and fertility. Since the first successful in vitro fertilization (IVF) in 1978, ten million children have been born through ART. Unimaginable advances have been made. Male factor issues can now be treated by injecting a sperm directly into an egg. Age-related female infertility can be managed by transferring eggs from a younger woman. Egg freezing can be done for fertility preservation with cancer and other patients. Preimplantation genetic testing can diagnose diseases. These are but a few of the medical breakthroughs that help patients on their path to parenthood.

But the benefits of ART are not without their costs. These advances stretch patients financially, physically, and emotionally. The stress of infertility is well documented, as is the stress of treatment. Many patients experience symptoms of depression and anxiety. As treatment intensifies, the distress in infertility patients often increases. This may contribute to patients leaving treatment prematurely, which therefore lowers pregnancy rates. As a physician who has spent a lifetime working in this field, I believe we have an obligation to treat our patients' emotional as well as medical needs. In fact, treating the former will enhance our ability to treat the latter.

Holistic medical care considers medical procedures, pharmaceuticals, and self-care to be necessary components. From this perspective, emotional well-being and lifestyle behaviors comprise an essential part in treatment. When patients practice mind-body skills, make positive changes in their lifestyles, and obtain social support, this facilitates and enhances treatment.

We are extremely fortunate to be able to partner with experienced providers such as Dr. Janetti Marotta. She has helped thousands of patients seek parenthood from every family-building option available. What she has learned from her own experience with infertility and from her work with others brings messages of hope, strength, and possibility. She has thought hard about the lessons learned from the experience of infertility and how to develop the resilience to stay the course and realize one's dream of parenthood. Dr. Marotta has written this mindfulness-based program book regarding fertility to help patients develop inner strength to face the challenges of treatment. We hope patients will use the mindfulness and compassion practices found in this book while under care.

David Adamson, MD, FRCSC, FACOG, FACS
Medical Director, Palo Alto Medical Foundation Fertility Physicians
Clinical Professor ACF, Stanford University School of Medicine
Associate Clinical Professor, UCSF School of Medicine

Preface

Welcome to *A Fertile Path: Guiding the Journey with Mindfulness and Compassion*. Here you will find a treasury of mindfulness teachings, practices, and exercises to cultivate your inner resources and meet the challenges of your fertility journey with a clear mind and open heart.

Our minds have the power to influence our health both physically and emotionally. Emotions are physiological processes that, just like yoga or diabetes, can affect our physical health. Mindfulness, or nonjudgmental present-moment awareness, is now a vital component of medical treatment for a wide range of health challenges. Mindfulness programs in education, workplace, and community settings are increasingly emerging as a way to decrease stress, enhance skill development, and promote physical and emotional well-being. More than a stress-reduction technique or self-improvement plan, mindfulness is a *way of being* that meets whatever trial or tribulation life presents. This book fosters mindfulness and compassion to complement fertility and its treatment, lessen the burden of your challenge, and move in the direction of health and healing.

Stress and fertility are intimately related. There is now a sufficient amount of high-quality research to conclude a positive relationship between lower emotional distress from effective psychological interventions and increased pregnancy rates. Optimizing self-care optimizes medical care. From a whole-person perspective, fertility treatment must include not only medicines and procedures but also self-nurturance.

Infertility represents a life crisis and is typically experienced as one of the most difficult situations ever encountered. Above all, we know infertility is stressful and wholly consuming. The demands of infertility impact the most important areas of our lives: our relationships, our careers, our finances, and especially our sense of self. We assume we can have children whenever we choose, that procreation is a birthright. When infertility challenges this assumption, the inability to father a child or become pregnant becomes our personal catastrophe.

Choosing a mind-body approach can feel overwhelming when you are already swamped by the costs and strains of fertility treatments. In fact, mind-body practices help you make more room for yourself—they create energy for the demands of living. The investment you make in caring for yourself is tiny compared to the rewards you will reap.

Congratulations for finding the courage to create time and space to work toward healing yourself. Accepting "what is" may seem impossible, but you begin by acknowledging it, as acknowledgment enables you to "befriend" whatever unwelcomed emotion comes knocking at your door. By giving yourself the opportunity to feel what is true, including the sorrow, and learning to take care of yourself with mindfulness practices, you can create a space where you can heal.

Here in the Western world, we often believe that if something is wrong, it's our fault. You have probably heard, "If you'd just relax, you'd get pregnant!" While the mind-body approach acknowledges that stress and fertility are related, *it does not imply you are in control of what you cannot control*. Mind-body medicine is about taking charge by taking care of your whole self.

The practices in *A Fertile Path* are mindfulness-based. Dr. Jon Kabat-Zinn, renowned mindfulness teacher, researcher, and Mindfulness-Based Stress Reduction (MBSR) Program founder, defines meditation—the heart of mindfulness—like this: "More than anything else, I have come to see meditation as an act of love, an inward gesture of benevolence and kindness toward ourselves and toward others, a gesture of the heart that recognizes our perfection even in our obvious imperfection, with all our shortcomings, our wounds, our attachments, our vexations, and our persistent habits of unawareness" (2005, 69).

*The practices included here invite you to
remember who you are at the center of yourself.*

Before the crisis of infertility resolves, you may experience depression, anxiety, and social isolation. Comments meant to be helpful—such as "Why don't you just adopt?"—can feel minimizing and hurtful. Receiving an invitation to one more baby shower can create an internal conflict: Do you support your friend or protect yourself?

Learning coping skills aimed at maximizing self-nurturance can help you deal with these difficult encounters and situations. Rather than avoiding people, places, or feelings, you can develop strategies that are proactive and helpful. Consciously choosing how to respond gives you permission to say yes and no.

These teachings and exercises offer understanding, clarity, and strength to help you through your journey. You are invited to use these mindfulness-based practices regularly; this will deepen your meditation practice and strengthen your trust in yourself. Mindfulness and trust are the antidotes to fear.

I honor the inward gesture of benevolence and kindness you are taking toward yourself in cultivating your own healing resources.

*May you receive and accept this invitation
to make room for yourself,
to be whole, to trust yourself,
and to travel on a fertile path.*

Acknowledgments

To the caring, accepting family I was born into and my cherished, beautiful family that emerged, proving the Beatles right: "All You Need Is Love!" Special gratitude to my husband, Steve, for sharing and growing together on our fertility journey; to my children Prairie and Tenaya for making room in their childhoods while we pursued many family-building options; and to Cheyenne, our gift from the long and windy road of infertility that led her to us. If there is but one lesson I am grateful to have learned, it's that only when you *let go* do you find what you are truly looking for.

To all fertility patients with whom I've worked: I have a deep appreciation for your courage and presence of mind to look within and seek to find your way. It's been my honor to shepherd you on your own personal journeys.

My highest regard to David Adamson, MD, for the immense impact he has made on the field of infertility and his commitment to treating both the medical and emotional needs of patients. It's been my honor to lead the mind-body program he founded in his center and to have his support in the partnership of this book by ARC Fertility (Advanced Reproductive Care, Inc.). Regards also to Gitte Pope, who helped form this partnership there.

Gratitude is extended to the mind-body team at Palo Alto Medical Foundation Fertility Physicians for their support in integrating this mindfulness-based model, the following individuals in particular: Lynn Brokenshire, MA, LMFT, leader of many of our mind-body programs and support services; Shannon Hare, our initial internal coordinator, who helped with the establishment and growth of the program; Kathleen McKenna, our current internal coordinator, who keeps the program up and running; Mary Abusief, MD, our physician sponsor who advocates for our program and an integrated approach into the practice; and the many staff members who have supported the mind-body program by helping steer patients toward it since its inception. Recognition to leaders in the field of mind-body treatment for fertility, most notably Alice Domar, PhD, and her groundbreaking research and approach.

Appreciation to Lee Ann O'Neal, LMFT, for the book's cover design; my daughter, Cheyenne Woodward, for the chapter head illustrations; Renee Burgard, LCSW, for recommendations on the Preface and collegial guidance in mindfulness; my husband, Steve Woodward, for his advice in the writing and preparation of the manuscript; Leslie Woodward, for her editing of the initial chapters; Joel Pitney, for his expertise in launching this book; Ari Karistenfeld, for his involvement in web design and outreach; and the CreateSpace team for their editorial and project assistance.

Fundamentally, all mindfulness teachings and practices found in this book can be traced back over twenty-five hundred years ago to the time of Buddha. Buddhist teachings show how we get stuck and how to break free; the Path of Liberation points the way. To the Buddha and his teachings, I give eternal gratitude. And to those extraordinary teachers today who inspire with their wisdom, deep appreciation is extended, especially His Holiness the Dalai Lama, Vietnamese Buddhist monk Thich Nhat Hanh, Mindfulness-Based Stress Reduction (MBSR) founder Jon Kabat-Zinn, and American Buddhist nun Pema Chodron. Appreciation also to such notable insight-meditation teachers as Jack Kornfield, Sharon Salzberg, Tara Brach, and Sylvia Boorstein, as well as my MBSR mentor Bob Stahl and meditation teacher Shaila Catherine.

Gratitude to my Dharma peer-support group for the ongoing encouragement in bringing mindfulness into our lives: Liz Trom, Nisar Shaikh, Cindi Crow-Urgo, Paul Ries, Shirley Kwok, and Humaira Mahi, also to all Insight Meditation South Bay sangha members for the support gained by being part of a community.

To those near and far, from ancient times to present day: family, friends, mentors, colleagues, patients, group members, teachers, and masters—I bow to you all!

Introduction

A Fertile Path can be used as a personal "midwife" to guide you through the difficult labor of your fertility journey. The mindfulness and compassion practices are sequentially based steps that will help shift you from the coping mechanism of control to awareness as a *way of being*.

To learn how to guide your fertility journey with mindfulness and compassion, I will introduce you to the formal practices of meditation in stillness and movement and the informal practices of applying mindfulness to everyday life. Throughout the book, you will cultivate such qualities as acceptance, nonjudgment, patience, and openness to stay the course of your fertility journey and realize your dream of parenthood. There are journaling and mindful-inquiry activities and exercises for exploration and discovery.

The teachings and practices begin with the foundational practice of mindfulness of the breath and body to turn on the relaxation response and anchor to the present moment. I will introduce you to the practice of yoga, which teaches that the breath exerts a powerful influence on the body and mind and imparts a sequence of poses believed by some yoga experts to be beneficial for fertility. I will also familiarize you with chi kung, a practice used in China to complement fertility by the cultivation of energy through slow, graceful movements and controlled deep breathing. You will find the lessons you learn in mindful-awareness practices apply to the lessons you learn in life itself.

I will teach you how to work with thoughts skillfully so you can detach from chronic, negative thought patterns and invite wholesome thoughts to emerge as well as how to hold emotions caringly so they can soften and dissolve in a wide and spacious heart. To increase your capacity to love yourself and others, compassion practices provide the courage and nurturance to meet challenging interpersonal situations, find balance in your intimate relationships, rejuvenate fertile health, and open to family-building options.

This book can be used as a ten-week individualized program or a peer-led group program. If you are a professional specializing in the field of fertility and have a mindfulness practice, you can use this book in your counseling service or in a professionally led group. The program has been developed over the last eight years and is highly rated by the hundreds of women and men who have participated in it, whether that be as group participants or counseling patients. While participating in this program onsite is ideal, I believe this book will help you approach your experience with balance and resilience. Connecting with a community that offers mindfulness programs can strengthen and deepen your mindfulness practice and participating in an infertility support program can help you feel not so alone in your challenge. In the back of the book, you will find resources that I have provided for you.

Spending a week on each of the ten chapters helps establish and maintain a daily mindfulness practice, integrate the teachings, and cultivate qualities along the way. Finding a consistent time and place for your formal practice strengthens its growth. Each chapter presents a formal and informal practice described in full, and weekly practice logs at the end of each chapter help track progress. Exercises are included to support the teachings, and recording your experience in a designated journal is recommended to deepen understanding. To listen to guided meditations that complement the formal practices covered in each chapter, go to www.janettimarotta.com/meditations.

Most importantly, move through this book at a pace that is right for you. By going through *A Fertile Path*, your own birthing process will unfold as you uncover your true nature—whole and complete already.

⌒Ɂᴵᐟ⋋

My Journey

My infertility story began in 1988, the year my husband, Steve, and I were married. During a pregnancy conceived two months into the marriage, we learned through amniocentesis of a genetic defect. We consulted experts all over the United States, Canada, and Britain and thought of little else for the scant two weeks we had to make the biggest decision of our lives. Finally, through fear, confusion, anguish, and love, we made the decision to terminate the pregnancy. Nothing prepared us for what came next.

First, there was one miscarriage, then a second, and then, at the age of thirty-nine, I was diagnosed with premature ovarian failure. With my follicle stimulating hormone (FSH) level at fifty-four, we attempted IVF, working under the assumption that "menopause was imminent" (eight years later, it was still imminent). Predictably, our one fertilized egg did not lead to a pregnancy. Over the next two years, we underwent one donor IVF cycle with my generous sister and four fresh cycles with our lovely donor.

As excruciating as these IVF cycles already were, two were further complicated by the fact that I became naturally pregnant at the same time. Tragically, these pregnancies also ended in miscarriage. My body was not able to sustain a growing life. After further soul searching, we turned next to both adoption and surrogacy, pursued simultaneously. After losing one potential adoption, we were matched with Leann, the woman who would turn out to be the family surrogate for our daughter Cheyenne.

At our first meeting, via telephone, Leann and I both felt like we were "falling in love." We talked for two hours, sharing amazing similarities and feeling instant connection. We first met in person with our husbands and later met Leann's daughter, parents, brother, and friends. We could not imagine a more auspicious beginning.

Five months of inseminations later, though, we were afraid we were confronting yet another failure. Even under the best of conditions, surrogacy can be difficult. Leann, it turned out, had polycystic ovaries, and the doctor's recommendation was Clomid. Leann was not comfortable taking this drug and came very close to bowing out of our shared endeavor.

Over the four years of infertility, I tried every means available to treat my physical, emotional, and spiritual being. I left my position in the psychiatry department at Stanford and began a private practice, which afforded more control over my schedule and caseload. As a patient myself, I engaged in individual, couples, and family therapy. I tried acupuncture, along with a prescribed acupuncture "exorcism" and medicinal teas. I went on several Vision Quests, eventually became a Vision Quest guide, and joined a Buddhist zendo.

Finally, I found "home" on an East-West spiritual path. I became able to release my guilt and more fully grieve for our lost babies. With fellow spiritual seekers, I left on a pilgrimage to India the very day of our fifth and perhaps last artificial insemination cycle with Leann. Steve and I said good-bye at the San Francisco Airport as he left for the cycle in Los Angeles and I left for the pilgrimage in India.

On the very first day of our pilgrimage, we visited Chattapur Temple during the celebration of Lord Shiva, god of destruction and rebirth. A fire started in the makeshift gathering hall, and within minutes, the flimsy structure was ablaze. We barely escaped with our lives.

Half a world away, another spark took hold. In Indian tradition, fire is known as the purifier because it loosens the *chitta* or karma that holds us back. I believe it was during this fire, or very near to it in time, when the conception of our baby occurred. When I met my husband one month later at the San Francisco airport, he was wearing a big pillow under his shirt!

The remaining eight months of our pregnancy were a time of immense growth for me. Despite my awe and anticipation, I also experienced feelings of loss, jealousy, and fear. After all, someone else was doing something so personal for me (and my husband), something I could no longer do. Each step in the process created new issues. However, at this point in the fertility experience, I was able to translate these feelings into lessons and opportunities. Each time I experienced a distressing emotion, I witnessed myself constricted by fear. In response, I opened to the pain and ultimately found trust, gratitude, and nurturance. With each ebb and flow, each contraction and expansion, my ability to stay open and accepting became my own birthing experience.

In my attempts to cope with infertility, I accidentally came upon a treasure chest of mind-body practices, often where I least expected. My major coping strategy of trying harder and eventually succeeding was no longer "how my world worked." Infertility is a crisis not only because of its effects on every area in life but also because the way you typically deal with difficulty no longer works. My major coping strategy of control, or trying harder to succeed, only resulted in a further sense of failure and hopelessness.

It is said we only change when we have more to lose by not changing. Reaching this juncture is what turned my crisis into opportunity, as I grew in ways otherwise out of my reach. Through awareness and cultivating qualities of acceptance, nonjudgment, patience, trust, and compassion, I became able to engage in the process and "let things be." I could then open to possibility and invite in all family-building options. I began to believe I would have a child.

As a psychologist, my specialty in infertility grew from my own personal journey and has been nurtured and strengthened through mindfulness. This book and my work with those challenged by infertility is drawn from my own personal experience, my professional work with patients over the years, and my mindfulness practice. My hope is that you will find these teachings as healing and transformative as I have.

Cheyenne is now twenty-three years old, and not a day has passed that I have not felt gratitude. We love Leann and her family, and all of us feel blessed by the experience we shared, difficult and expensive as it was. For three years after Cheyenne's conception, my FSH decreased to five. During this time, a woman remarked to me, "Now you can have your own child." What she didn't realize, and what I came to realize through this journey, is I do have my own child. I understand things in a different way now. Infertility, and its resolution through surrogacy, has taught me that Cheyenne, like every child, is a child of the universe and a gift from beyond (Marotta 2013, 12–13).

One

Turning on the Relaxation Response

Every bell has a crack in it. That's how the light gets in.

—Leonard Cohen

The Paradox of Infertility

Though infertility is a medical condition, it often becomes much more: a challenge to your identity at its core. As an infertile person, you internalize *Webster*'s definition: *not fertile or productive:* BARREN, synonym STERILE. Here lies the central paradox: How is it that, in this very quest to bring new life into the world, you bring so little life of your own?

Believing this definition of infertility is really scary, so you do what your instincts tell you to do—*hide or run!* The possibility that the fertility doctor might give an unwanted diagnosis can be so terrifying that you may perpetually delay the appointment or perhaps never go. Conversely, when you pursue treatment, you may not be able to stop, setting an addictive course that leads to increasingly lower probabilities of success. You race against time to find the *one good egg*, feeling you're not just running to become pregnant, but literally *running for your life*.

Paradoxically, those very qualities you need most are least accessible. You assume, judge, mistrust, strive, and become impatient. You are fixated on how it "should be" and are trapped between grasping and pushing away. You engage in self-blame and criticism. Ultimately, you believe you have only yourself to blame. It is easy to give in to *Webster*'s definition and see yourself as broken. It then becomes a natural compulsion to fix yourself, believing that only when you've reached your goal can you feel whole.

For most people, the more prolonged the struggle with infertility, the greater the costs. Over time, infertility can erode relationships—with your partner, friends, relatives, and the community at large. You can become a stranger to yourself, with traumatic consequences to your home and work life and your physical and emotional health.

Why does infertility lead to such alienation? We often feel that bringing a child into our primary relationship is the ultimate affirmation of shared affection, and bringing a child into the world can feel like our one true connection to the progress of humanity and the stream of time. Infertility undermines these assumptions about ourselves; it questions our place in the world.

The repeated failure to create a child together can become disaffirming to your central relationship. It reignites issues you may have assumed were re-solved or magnifies issues you may have considered insignificant. Rather than sharing in a joint venture, partners often struggle with each other and split into opposing camps. As infertility drags on month after month, couples have less and less to give one another, when what they need is more and more. This is but one of the many paradoxes of infertility.

Additional paradoxes await in other key areas of life:

Family, friends, and community. You often experience innocent comments from those personally unfamiliar with infertility, however close to you they may be in other areas of life, as insensitive and uncaring. The joyful advent of a friend's pregnancy, even a friend who has struggled to conceive, can make your heart sink. The mall full of baby strollers becomes an emotional minefield. These sensitivities can lead you to isolate yourself. Despite an ever-increasing need for support and understanding, you may feel the urge to retreat further and further away from help.

Work. As you pour effort into demanding infertility treatments, your work life can become unmanageable. Your career is threatened at a time when you need it as a source of self-esteem and income. You need to slow down even as you are expected to try harder.

Time. Infertility is often a race against your biological clock. You must make difficult decisions under time pressures whose consequences may be lifelong. How can you be patient while needing to move forward quickly? How can you slow down when expected to move faster and try harder?

Decisions. Advanced reproductive technology (ART) gives an ever-expanding range of choices in efforts to bring a child into your family, and you are required to understand, in depth, what these choices mean. A year in fertility treatment is like a year in graduate school. You need to understand reproductive biology, endocrinology, family law, contracts, torts, international law, perhaps another language—and most of it in whatever spare time you have at night. The wealth of options can distract you from the reality that these decisions must be made from the heart. Ultimately, moving through infertility is not only about knowing ART but also about knowing who you are. It is about knowing many things, but also one thing.

Control. A nearly universal experience of infertility is the feeling of being *out of control.* The world is broken. What has always worked no longer does. Trying harder brings greater failure. You are in a fight for your life, but you do not know the rules. At every turn, you are asked to let go, let go, let go. At the same time, the secret to relinquishing control can be found only within your-self. Jungians say, "God enters through the wound."

The Final Paradox. Infertility is a catastrophe in every sense of the word. Yet it is the very struggle of infertility and its diminishing of reserves in every domain of life that can ultimately replenish and further you. It requires you to look for happiness not on the outside but on the inside. The continual con-tractions—through withdrawal, resentment, fear, and panic—make you thirst for expansion: trust, acceptance, peace, and finally liberation.

Everyone seeks happiness, and at this very moment when happiness seems lost, the human spirit will fight hardest to find where it lives. The final para-dox is that infertility is inevitably a birthing process. The labor is difficult and frightening, and we resist, but the process carried through brings forth a new spirit in all who are open to it.

The Paradox of Mindfulness

More than a stress-reduction technique, mindfulness is a *way of being*—a meth-od of meeting what Taoists call "the ten thousand joys and the ten thousand sorrows" inherent in the human experience. Mindfulness cultivates the quali-ties you most need, such as acceptance, patience, and trust, and transforms the most insurmountable obstacles and plights into challenges and opportunities for growth. Mindfulness does not change or take away the situation—in this case infertility—but provides the vehicle for you to *become* the change itself.

With awareness as the midwife, mindfulness teaches you to relax, release, and let go: to breathe through every contraction of holding tight on to what you want or trying to get rid of what you don't want and to open to the un-folding process of life. Through repeated practice, you learn *resistance* is how you get stuck and *acceptance* is how you break free.

Mindfulness welcomes what is here, regardless what it is. At every junc-ture, you are invited to *be with* what is happening. You learn to relinquish control not by trying to change the situation, or even yourself, but rather by changing your *relationship* to what is occurring and working from here. As you do this, you cultivate the cornerstone quality of acceptance: a state of open receptivity, a willingness to *turn toward* that which you resist. Paradoxically, when you accept things as they are, you are better able to assess the situation, find your strength, make wise choices, and take wholesome actions.

There is so much in life you cannot control, and your efforts to try to change what you don't like only intensify the problem. When you let go of control, insecurity, and rigidity, you open, release, and let things be. You are shifting from the coping mechanism of control—trying to change what is—to acceptance by being with what is.

Mindfulness rests at the center of Buddhist psychology. In contrast to Western psychology, Buddhist psychology finds wisdom in paradox. For this very reason, mindfulness uses paradox to meet life's challenges and becomes the perfect antidote for the paradoxical land mines infertility presents.

Mindfulness is often likened to driving on ice. When the road is icy, your natural instinct to stop spinning out of control is to turn away from the skid. But the way to maintain control is by turning into the skid. Mindfulness teaches you to turn toward discomfort rather than away from it. This is the way to break free.

To practice mindfulness is to know and see things as they are—to observe the arising and passing of thoughts, emotions, and experience. It is an invitation to be fully alive and awake to your own experience. Mindfulness creates a sense of spaciousness so the mind can be open and able to contain all things without limitation. Mindfulness embraces an attitude of curiosity, approaching situations without judgment. It is a way to open the mind to exploration and discovery of one's deeper self. This spacious and curious mind cultivates patience—understanding that some situations unfold in their own time, without your control. You understand it is not the destination but the journey that matters. As Vietnamese mindfulness teacher, monk, and peace activist Thich Nhat Hanh says: "There is no way to happiness, happiness is the way."

Mindfulness starts from the perspective that you are whole and complete already, regardless of flaws or imperfections. In contrast to the Western notion of original sin, Buddhist psychology is based on the concept of *original goodness*: your essential nature—your *Buddha nature*—is good and pure.

Proceeding from this vantage point gives you freedom from the bondage of inadequacy and insecurity.

The entry to mindfulness is through the vehicle of meditation. Through meditation, you learn to anchor *attention* to what is called an object, such as the breath, and set an *intention* to stay with this object. Because the mind naturally wanders, you notice the habits of the restless mind. You become aware of how thoughts create stories that lead down dark and endless alleys, such as "I'll never get pregnant" or "I'm a failure." You also recognize thoughts without letting them define who you are. You learn to move between effort and surrender, simultaneously taking intentional steps while becoming part of life's dynamic flow. Grasping this paradox is an important turning point on the mindful journey.

Mindfulness challenges assumptions about *who* you are and *why* you are doing *what* you are doing. Through mindful inquiry, you look deeply into such questions as these:

"Is infertility the obstacle, or is fertility the challenge?"
"Is infertility happening to me or *for* me?"
"Is my true longing pregnancy or parenthood?"
"Is infertility the loss of a dream or a dream not awakened?"

It's not about following the prescription that leads from point *A* to point *B*; rather, it is answering the invitation to *drop into your heart*—to come full circle on the wheel of paradox that starts with loving yourself just as you are and ends with loving yourself just as you are. Through this gateway, you give birth to yourself.

Taking the First Step

We apply the key principle of original goodness to the first step on your journey to fertility. When you focus on what's wrong, you strive to compensate or fill the void in your desperate attempt to be OK—in this case, fertile. But when you focus on what is *not wrong*, you start from the perspective of accepting yourself as you are, with all your inadequacies and insecurities, including the fact of your infertility. Paradoxically, it is not until you accept yourself for who you are that you are free to change.

As you open the door to original goodness, you invite the possibility of *original fertility*: you are already rich, fruitful, productive, and creative. Begin by settling your mind and opening your heart, and prepare to uncover the deep intention that led you to this book. Settle the body in a comfortable upright, relaxed, and alert position and gently close your eyes. Notice the breath naturally occurring. As you bring light attention to the breath, notice the rhythm of the in-breath and the out-breath. Imagine your eyes dropping down from their sockets so you are *seeing* from your heart. Visualize breathing into and out from your heart. The heart knows no limits as each breath opens and expands its reach.

Ask yourself: "What is the deep motivation that brings me here right now? What is something I appreciate about myself that can further me on this journey?" Rather than seeking the answer, let the answer find you. When ready, slowly open your eyes. Affirm your intention and attribute that emerged. Do you have even a small sense that you are the one you have been looking for?

⌒╱╲╲⌐

Stress, Fertility, and the Mind–Body Connection

The fact that infertility and its overwhelming effects is a crisis is supported by studies that have found levels of depression and anxiety in women diagnosed with infertility equal to those in patients diagnosed with cancer, HIV, and heart disease (Domar, Zuttermeister, and Friedman 1993). In a study that interviewed women before their first fertility clinic visits, 40.2 percent met criteria for a psychiatric disorder, as compared with an average prevalence of 3 percent (Chen et al. 2004), and another study reported infertility to be the most stressful experience in many women's lives (Freeman et al. 1985).

A review of the literature (Eugster and Vingerhoets 1999) concludes that beyond a doubt IVF is physically and emotionally stressful for women and partners alike, with anxiety and depression being the most common reactions to treatment. Moreover, psychological distress is correlated with treatment termination (Domar et al. 2010). In a recent study with four hundred women aged forty years old and younger, highly stressed women were 40 percent less likely to conceive during their ovulation windows (Akhter et al. 2016). So what is the stress-fertility connection, and how can you actively engage to move in the direction of health and healing?

To understand how stress harms the body, we need to look at the autonomic nervous system. Operating at a subconscious level, the autonomic nervous system controls many functions of the internal organs and glands, including hormone secretion. It is central to our ability to feel and experience emotions. Because emotions are both mental expressions generated by the brain and physiological states that affect our health, it is the autonomic nervous system that connects our brain, body, and heart.

The autonomic nervous system has two branches: the sympathetic nervous system and the parasympathetic nervous system. The sympathetic system controls the stress response, also known as the fight-or-flight response. The stress response tells the body to take immediate action. When confronted by danger, the sympathetic nervous system induces shallow, rapid breathing.

When triggered, stress hormones—adrenalin and cortisol—are pumped to every organ; endorphins surge to numb pain; heart rate, blood pressure, and respiration rise to mobilize muscle and movement; and blood vessels constrict where energy is not needed (skin and body core) while others enlarge where energy is needed (brain and limbs). It is the stress response that enabled us to run from the saber-toothed tiger and remain on the planet today. Once danger passes, the body returns to normal within a short amount of time.

But what happens under chronic stress conditions? In today's society, we experience many fear-inducing situations throughout the day, beginning with the sound of the alarm clock; if a person has a chronic medical condition, such as infertility, stress increases exponentially. But the brain cannot distinguish between what is life threatening and what is emotionally threatening. Lurking behind nearby bushes are "demon" tigers—internal voices that frighten us with roaring thoughts of doom and gloom (Marotta 2013, 17). The body stays on crisis mode, under a constant heightened level of response. Chronic stress can cause a host of ailments, including the following: high blood pressure, which damages blood vessels; muscle tension, which produces muscle tightness or spasms;

a suppressed immune system, which impacts the ability to fight disease; and a suppressed digestive system, which increases stomach acid and produces irritable bowel syndrome.

While the physiological mechanism has not been determined, stress also appears to suppress fertility, which makes it harder to conceive. Because infertility is itself a chronic stressor, the stress response remains activated. From this defensive position, your automatic reaction is to protect yourself and operate from *me versus them* mode. Chest breathing becomes the default—short, fast, shallow breaths that turn on the stress response. This conditioned breathing is like putting your foot on the gas pedal. Your body is revved up. Over time, your body begins to wear out, and the toll you pay is on your physical health and emotional well-being.

But what if the relationship to the stressor changes? What if the mind is able to tell the body, "Don't worry; it's going to be OK?" Through examination of psychosocial interventions that focus on stress reduction to improve pregnancy rate, the last twenty years have now produced enough high-quality studies to sufficiently demonstrate the power of the mind-body connection in fertility. A recent meta-analysis of thirty-nine qualified studies found not only decreased symptoms of psychological distress for the intervention groups but also increased pregnancy rates (Frederiksen et al. 2015). In fact, women in the intervention groups were twice as likely to become pregnant than those in the control groups. The higher pregnancy rates found in the groups receiving the psychosocial interventions that reduce infertility-related distress support the hypothesis that stress impacts fertility.

Exercise: Infertility Stress Test

Below are emotional symptoms common to infertility. Complete this *infertility stress test* to see how many symptoms relate to you. When challenged by fertility, anxious and depressed symptoms are at par for the course, but it's important to know if you're clinically depressed so you can get help. To determine whether you have depression, you might want to start by taking a free screening tool offered by Mental Health America at www.mentalhealthamerica.net/mental-health-screening-tools.

I feel like a failure because I'm unable to become pregnant or carry a pregnancy.	yes	no
I'm afraid I may never give birth or hold a pregnancy.	yes	no
I don't feel the support I need from my partner.	yes	no
I feel jealous or sad when I hear that someone else is pregnant.	yes	no
I avoid friends and family members who are pregnant or have babies.	yes	no
I'm having difficulty making decisions on how to deal with infertility.	yes	no
I feel I'm being punished.	yes	no
I resent how infertility is impacting my life.	yes	no
I feel my life is on hold.	yes	no
I feel overwhelmed or a loss of control over my life.	yes	no
I'm hurt by comments like "just relax" that minimize the difficulty of infertility.	yes	no
I experience less pleasure and enjoyment.	yes	no
My sex life is suffering.	yes	no
My career is being impacted by infertility.	yes	no
My sleep is disturbed by thoughts related to infertility.	yes	no

The Relaxation Response

The parasympathetic nervous system controls the relaxation response. As with the stress response, a change in the breath triggers the relaxation response. Instead of the rapid, shallow breath that sets off the fight-or-flight urge, deep abdominal breathing induces the relaxation response by stimulating the vagus nerve. This adept wandering nerve travels between the brain and most organs, signaling the body to slow down and relax.

Repeated studies show that relaxation and meditation reduce stress by lowering the heart rate, blood pressure, and levels of stress hormones, while enhancing the immune function. Adverse health symptoms decrease, including insomnia, hypertension, and migraines. The increased pregnancy rate from psychosocial intervention studies has helped in establishing this link between stress and fertility.

The long, slow, deep breathing from the abdomen is called natural breathing because this is how we breathed when we were born. Natural breathing is like putting your foot on the brake pedal: your nervous system cools down, your body functions with greater ease, and your brain operates in a peaceful state—from *we* mode—a state of wholeness and connection to others. You only need to reactivate your memory to return to natural breathing and utilize what Andrew Weil calls "the master key to self healing."

Breath work is centuries old and progressively recommended by health-care providers as an important stress-reduction technique and way to positively affect health:

> Indeed, of all the approaches that I have recommended to people for improving health, the single technique that I get the most positive feedback about is breath work. Over and over again I am impressed with the power of working with breath as a technique to improve various conditions and to boost general well-being. I feel very strongly as a result of these experiences that proper breathing is a master key to good health. (Weil 2005, 12)

You begin this journey as an active participant in your health and well-being by learning how to *turn off* the stress response and *turn on* the relaxation response with abdominal breathing. As you gain experience on how to lower stress and care for your whole self, a safe and quiet refuge will emerge. You come to understand the wisdom of this saying by psychologist and founder of gestalt therapy, Fritz Perls: "Fear is only excitement without the breath."

Exercise: Belly Breathing

Begin this exercise by lying on your back. This relaxes the belly and enables you to most easily determine your breathing pattern. Place one hand on your belly and the other hand on your chest. Now gently close your eyes.

Notice if the hand on your belly is moving higher on the inhalation and lower on the exhalation than the hand on your chest. If so, you are breathing from your abdomen. The diaphragm is a muscle that separates the chest from the abdominal cavity, and when the breath is long, slow, and deep, the diaphragm moves down when you inhale, causing your belly to rise, and moves up when you exhale, causing your belly to fall.

The belly appears like a balloon, gently filling with air as you inhale and emptying its air as you exhale. As this filling and emptying occurs, oxygen and carbon dioxide move in and out. The diaphragm is massaging the heart, lungs, and abdominal organs as the lungs, chest, back, and belly are rhythmically opening and closing. Breathing is deep, slow, quiet, and smooth.

To more finely tune in to whether you are properly engaged in abdominal breathing, be sure it is the inhalation and not the exhalation that causes your belly to expand—otherwise you are reversing your breathing. If the hand on your chest is moving higher than the hand on your belly, breathing is shallow and you're breathing from your chest. Notice too if the inhalation is longer than the exhalation (if not, you are overbreathing), if breathing is smooth (there's no "catch" between the in-breath and out-breath), and if breathing is from your nose (as opposed to from your mouth).

To invite the breath to slow and deepen, try this visualization exercise. As you're lying down with your eyes closed, feel your body supported by the earth. Imagine yourself lying in the shade on a soft, sandy, beautiful beach on a warm, clear day. In the near distance is the sound of gentle waves massaging the shore—waves coming in, waves going out. Inhaling, your belly expands as you hear the gentle wave wash onto shore. Exhaling, your belly deflates as the wave whispers back to sea. Your belly gently rises on the wave of the in-breath and falls on the wave of the out-breath. Follow the breath for its full duration as it matches with the slow, rhythmic wave coming into shore and going out to sea. Relax into the rhythmic healing massage of the breath.

When ready to leave the beach, slowly open your eyes. How did you feel? If you felt a sense of ease, rest, or relaxation, you were engaged in abdominal breathing. If not, with repeated practice your breath will slow and deepen on its own. Know you can return to this place of peace and calm throughout the day.

Staying the Course of Treatment

Since in vitro fertilization (IVF) was first successful in 1978, more than ten million babies have been born through assisted reproductive technology (ART). While IVF has brought the gift of parenthood to millions, it is not without its downside. Studies report a 23–65 percent IVF clinic dropout rate. It is therefore not surprising to expect a 50 percent dropout rate in a typical IVF clinic. Research indicates the primary reason for patients dropping out of treatment is not finances, diagnosis, or prognosis, but stress (Domar 2004). A systematic review of twenty-two studies on treatment dropout reinforces the conclusion that psychological issues (in particular treatment postponement, relational and personal factors, and psychological burden) are the greatest contributors (Gameiro, Boivin, and Verhaak 2012). Ending treatment after only one IVF cycle is more likely to occur in women found to be more depressed and anxious before beginning treatment (Smeenk et al. 2004). Ironically, the most distressed patients do not seek out psychological support (Boivin, Scanlan, and Walker 1999).

In a review that examined the use of stress management in fertility treatment (Campagne 2006), psychological interventions to reduce stress related to IVF were found to be generally effective, providing ample evidence that psychological distress impacts fertility and thus IVF outcomes. Campagne argues that IVF treatment should *start* with interventions to reduce stress. He suggests this could prepare the couple for an initial failed cycle, decrease the number of cycles, or make the more invasive procedures unnecessary.

Schlaff and Braverman (2015) introduced a series of articles that emphasized the importance of a more comprehensive model of mental health integration into infertility practice. In one of these articles, Domar (2015) strongly recommends a collaborative model because symptoms of anxiety and depression are unpleasant for the patient and challenging for the caregivers, distressed patients are more likely to terminate treatment, and psychological distress may be correlated with lower pregnancy rates. In a second article, Boivin and Gameiro (2015) reinforce how an integrated approach could reduce treatment burden stemming from a variety of sources, such as patient, clinic, and treatment.

In the University of Louisville's epidemiological study (Akhter et al. 2016) that confirms women's high stress reduces the likelihood of conceiving by 40 percent, Taylor asserts: "I hope the results of this study serve a wake-up call for both physicians and the general public that psychological health and well-being is just as important as other more commonly accepted risk factors such as smoking, drinking alcohol, or obesity when trying to conceive."

In order to acknowledge a fertility problem, accept a diagnosis, seek treatment, and develop a sound fertility plan, you must learn to manage stress in a healthy way. It is a well-known fact that people make better decisions after lowering stress, as it is only through a clear head and wise heart that real choices emerge. Reducing stress may not only improve your chance of a successful IVF outcome but also enable you to *stay the course* of treatment and realize your dream of parenthood.

Breath-Awareness Meditation

Meditation from every tradition uses breath awareness as a foundational practice. The breath is accessible in every moment—it's always with us and here for us. Meditation allows the breath to naturally slow and deepen, turning on the relaxation response. The breath anchors our attention to the present moment, away from past regret and guilt or future worry and fear. Because it stabilizes attention, it is the antidote to the wandering mind—known to be an unhappy mind. As a mind-training practice, meditation helps to not only lower stress but also develop insight and cultivate qualities to *stay the course*.

Formal Practice: Breath-Awareness Meditation

This beginning ten-minute breath-awareness meditation presents four meditation aides to stabilize attention. Try each option for one minute before moving to the next. For the remaining minutes, settle into the one that feels most *right* for you. Find a comfortable position, whether lying down on your back or sitting up with an erect, relaxed spine. Slowly close your eyes and take three deep, long breaths—inhaling life energy through the nostrils, exhaling tension away from the mouth. Now return to breathing at your own natural rhythm—inhaling and exhaling from your nostrils.

Count the breath. On the inhalation count one, and on the exhalation count two, until you've reached ten. Repeat. If you lose your place, start at one again.

Feel breath sensations. Feel the wave of the breath in the body, as the body lifts and expands on the inhalation and lowers and dissolves on the exhalation, or as the belly rises on the inhalation and falls on the exhalation. Repeat.

Touch and let go. Make a mental note "touch" as you lightly feel the breath on the inhalation. Make a mental note "let go" as you release tension in the body and mind on the exhalation. Repeat.

Mark the breath through touch. Place a rosary, mala, or beaded strand in your hand. After each breath cycle (in-breath, out-breath), move to the next bead. Alternatively, track the breath by touching one knuckle at a time. Continue.

When the mind wanders, as it will naturally do, gently but firmly escort the mind back to the breath. Know that every time the mind strays and you return to the breath, you are training the mind to stay put and be where you intend the mind to be, right in the present moment. Remember, it's the *coming back* that matters.

Use the practice log at the end of the chapter to record your experience. Note your preferred option, if you are able to stay with and return to the breath, and what you learned or how you benefitted. If you didn't engage in the practice or noticed some difficulty, note your challenges or what interfered. To listen to the guided meditation that complements this chapter's formal practice, go to www.janettimarotta.com/meditations.

Informal Practice: Belly-Breathing Awareness—Felt

This informal practice helps support abdominal breathing as your natural breathing pattern in everyday life through the use of a tactile reminder. Just as rosary beads, mala strands, or worry beads use physical sensation to anchor attention, this informal mindfulness practice called FELT relies on the sense of touch to "Feel Every Loving Touch" of the breath (Marotta 2013, 24–25). As you develop a positive, loving connection to the natural healing presence of the breath, you are connecting the body with the mind.

Cut small pieces of felt into the shape of a heart and then strategically place your FELTs in noticable places. You might choose to attach one to the back of your cell phone or laptop or keep one in your pocket or on your desk. When doing a FELT, take two to three slow, deep belly breaths. Use these breath reminders to nourish yourself throughout the day as you "feel every loving touch." Use the practice log at the end of the chapter to record your experience of the FELT practice. Note the influence of using this breath reminder to engage in abdominal breathing and connect with the nourishing touch of the breath.

Practice Log 1: Formal Practice—Breath Awareness Meditation

What did you learn/how did you benefit?   What were your challenges/what interfered?

DAY 1

DAY 2

DAY 3

DAY 4

DAY 5

DAY 6

DAY 7

Practice Log 1: Informal Practice—Belly Breathing Awareness - FELT
Note the influence of using this breath reminder to engage in abdominal breathing.

DAY 1

DAY 2

DAY 3

DAY 4

DAY 5

DAY 6

DAY 7

Two

ANCHORING TO THE BREATH

*Your vision will become clear only when you look into your
heart. Who looks outside, dreams. Who looks inside, awakens.*

—CARL JUNG

To deepen the connection to your natural healing and stabilizing power
of the breath, in chapter 2, I introduce you to mindfulness and the
foundational practice of mindfulness of the breath. Thich Nhat Hanh (2004,
track 1) describes the breath as the bridge that connects the mind to the body:
"The mind and body are re-unified and we're in one place…We stop the
thinking, and this is a miracle."

With the breath as your anchor to the present moment, you *train the brain*
to stay put—to not be seduced into rehashing the past or rehearsing the future
but rather to dwell in present-moment awareness where peace, strength, and
clarity reside and your whole and complete self can arise. In this chapter, I
invite you to use mindfulness as your guide, establish a meditation practice,

and develop a mindful road map to traverse the twists and turns of fertility treatment, including how to prepare for IVF, injections, and the pregnancy result call.

Why is mindfulness helpful for fertility? The cyclical nature of reproduction, with its monthly reminders, restimulates losses and failures of the past and generates fear and anxiety of the future, squeezing the present thin. Each monthly reminder emphasizes the passage of the time you've been trying to conceive. Mindfulness helps you stay in the present, maintain a neutral perspective, and not take on infertility as a *definition of self.* Mindfulness is knowing and seeing what is happening as it is occurring. Your mind and body are integrated so you can pay attention to what is actually present before you. The intensity of thoughts and overwhelmingness of emotions lessen, making it possible for new perspectives, possibilities, and strategies to emerge. You can develop such qualities as nonjudgment, bringing an attitude of neutral observation to any encounter, without labeling things as good or bad. You will find that this non-judgmental neutral lens will make all the difference in how you de-identify with infertility and experience the circuitous journey to parenthood.

Nowhere Is Now Here

Through our normal day, we do not spend much time at rest in the present moment. In fact, it's been found that the mind wanders 46.9 percent of the time. Thus, almost half of our time is spent practicing mindlessness, caught in automatic reactivity mode, not being where we actually are. As musician John Lennon said, "Life is what happens when we're busy making other plans."

We are living in what has been called an "epidemic of stress." We are too often critical with others, but even more often critical toward ourselves. We see the world through a lens of judgment that filters experience through what is wrong with ourselves or the situation. We find ourselves tilted ten degrees off-center: "If only I was thinner, had more money, was more successful, smarter, prettier..." The list goes on. We have shifted from being hunters and gatherers to shoppers looking for the best deal. And when we find it, we are too often disappointed or find that the pleasure doesn't seem to last very long. In being "human doers," we have forgotten to be human beings.

Not only do we trigger the stress response unconsciously multiple times a day as we worry about past and future in our drive for success, but we also intentionally stimulate the stress response as we equate "strain with gain." We then wonder why we are so exhausted, irritable, easily frustrated, and burned out. In fact, we learn more easily and perform better in a restful state, as the brain is more creative when we are peaceful.

The more you feel the ever-increasing tug of inadequacy from infertility, the more you relate to it with fear and trepidation. You hold tight on to fear, believing if you let go, you will never arrive at your destination. This creates a relationship of striving—trying harder and harder to succeed—rather than cultivating qualities to sustain you through the uphill trek.

Over twenty-five hundred years ago, Buddha looked at the nature of the mind and its relationship to suffering and freedom from suffering. "At the heart of Buddhist teachings is the recognition of the four noble truths: to understand the fact of suffering, to abandon the cause of suffering; to realize the end of suffering; to cultivate the way leading to the end of suffering" (Catherine 2008, 23).

Buddha showed the path to freedom from suffering through the vehicle of meditation, which informs the actions of skillful living. Buddha never presented himself as a messenger of divine power. When asked, "Are you a god, Buddha?" he replied, "No, I am awake!" Buddha was not a Buddhist; he was the awakened one.

The practice of mindfulness is to become awake, as only in the present can you truly come to know yourself. You let go of the delusion that you should be somewhere other than where you are: "there is truly nowhere to go, nothing to do, nothing to attain. You are already whole, already complete, just as you are—and that is perfect—for now—in the warm embrace of your own awareness" (Kabat-Zinn 2013, 574).

Mindfulness, MBSR, and Meditation

Mindfulness opens the door between a form of meditation developed in the time of the Buddha and mainstream medicine. Since 1989, when Kabat-Zinn made mindfulness the focus of an eight-week MBSR program, it has grown as a highly recognized treatment option and helped spur the "revolution of mindfulness" we have today. MBSR has an established track record for treating chronic pain, numerous medical conditions, and a range of stress-related disorders. Studies continue to demonstrate the beneficial effects of MBSR, mindfulness, and meditation on physical and mental health, relationships, skill development, and brain and immune system functioning.

In one such study by Dr. Richie Davidson and colleagues (2003) at the University of Wisconsin, employees at a high-tech company were randomly assigned to either an MBSR group or a wait-list control group. Initial MRI scans of all employees in the sample showed brain activity was "tipped to the right," meaning there was more brain activity toward the right hemisphere, where negative emotions predominately reside. By the end of the eight-week study, MRI scans for those employees attending the MBSR group showed brain activity had "tipped to the left," meaning there was more brain activity toward the left hemisphere, where positive emotions predominately reside. The control group, on the other hand, stayed "tipped to the right," the predominately negative emotion hemisphere of the brain. In addition, at the beginning of the study, employees were given flu vaccinations. The treatment group showed higher antibody levels at the end of the MBSR training compared to the control group, indicating an enhanced immune response. This study demonstrates how mindfulness practice can change the structure and function of the brain.

In a study at Stanford University by Philippe Goldin, PhD (2010), people with anxiety disorders participated in an eight-week MBSR program. Before and after the intervention, participants' brains were scanned in a functional MRI, a device which is often anxiety provoking even in the calmest of people. After the intervention, participants' amygdala, a region associated with stress and anxiety, showed decreased activation. Participants reported less anxiety and greater ability to stay calm.

The work of Antoine Lutz, PhD, and colleagues (2008b) at the University of Wisconsin shows how meditation activates regions of the brain critical for controlling attention. One study demonstrates how meditation can eventually reduce the effort it takes to focus attention. In another study, Dr. Lutz and colleagues (2008a) demonstrate how experienced meditators practicing compassion meditation showed a larger brain response in areas important for processing physical sensations and emotional responses. Meditation appears to impact a part of the brain involved in empathy.

In general, the two most prevalent kinds of meditation in the Buddhist tradition focus on concentration or insight. Concentration meditation focuses the mind on a single point, such as a mantra, phrase, or breath. Transcendental meditation, which settles attention on a mantra, is one example. Thoughts, emotions, bodily sensations, and senses are seen as distractions from the intention of sustaining the focus. This practice calms, stabilizes, and empowers the mind.

Insight meditation, or Vipassana, does not see thoughts, emotions, bodily sensations, or senses as distractions, but as part of the unfolding nature of experience to observe and relate to with nonjudgmental awareness. Vipassana, meaning "clear seeing," is an awareness practice that leads to insight and contributes to wisdom. At the center of insight meditation is the practice of mindfulness, the cultivation of clear, stable, and nonjudgmental awareness.

The Formal Practice

The formal mindfulness practice consists of meditation in both stillness and movement. Mindfulness meditation uses attention on an object to stay focused on the present moment with neutral observation and intention to stay fully present to your meditation so you can attain intimate awareness of what you're observing.

When learning how to meditate in the Vipassana, or insight meditation, tradition, instruction teaches you to focus on different objects of attention. Most commonly, the sequence consists of meditation on the breath, body, thoughts, and emotions. You learn to place "bare attention" on the object of attention—a single-minded awareness of what is actually happening in you and to you in the present moment. You come into intimate contact with sensations without needing to analyze, evaluate, or fix and notice how you are relating to the object of attention—whether you're relating with resistance (e.g., judgment) or acceptance (e.g., engagement). With attention comes the intention to stay with your object of attention. Psychiatrist and founder of interpersonal neurobiology Daniel Siegel (2010, 32) describes mindfulness meditation as having the capacity to *aim* and *sustain* attention with an *observant*, *objective*, and *open* stance.

Mindfulness meditation assumes that even with your best intention to stay with the breath, the mind will wander, as this is what the mind naturally does. It's easy to get caught in random thoughts and stories the mind weaves and lose what is foremost in your experience—the present moment. But a wandering mind is an unhappy mind, and in the training ground of meditation, you learn how to not be swept away by the undertows of the mind but stay on the present course. You can imagine the benefits of a stable mind when dealing with the compulsive thoughts and overwhelming emotions that infertility brings.

While meditating, every time the mind wanders, you simply make a mental note—"thinking"—and kindly escort yourself back to the object of attention. If your mind wanders five hundred times during one sitting, you get to practice *coming back* five hundred times. This is a valuable practice in and of itself. You are learning to get away from mindless chatter, to cultivate qualities that calm and sustain, and to shift from *control mode* to *awareness mode*.

Remember, mindfulness meditation is not about emptying the mind. This means there are no distractions. Thus, when sounds appear or body sensations are felt, rather than viewing sounds as a distraction or body sensations as an annoyance, they are seen as part of the unfolding nature of experience to observe and relate to with nonjudgmental awareness. Also, there is no such thing as a good or bad meditation. If you notice the mind straying away into "monkey mind" (the way monkeys swing from branch to branch), you learn how distracted the mind can be. Being aware of the habits of the mind is a fundamental part of the change process.

When you begin to see unwieldy habits of the mind while meditating, you begin to notice the force these habits have in everyday life. Understanding dysfunctional patterns helps shed light on how your way of living is not conducive for feeling at ease. You notice the way you grasp or avoid, pull or push—wanting to hold on to what you like and get rid of what you don't like. You become aware of how much effort you are expending and how ineffective this effort is. There is so much in life we can't control, and our efforts to change what we don't like paradoxically creates more of a problem. So, noticing this tendency is an important step in freeing yourself from suffering.

How you relate to the object of attention (e.g., breath, body, thoughts, or emotions) intersects with how you relate to life. As your awareness grows, you begin to see the cause-and-effect relationship in all things. Rather than attempting to change a situation, meditation teaches you to change your relationship to the situation, and this makes all the difference.

During meditation, you notice if you are relating to the object of attention with *acceptance* (feeling curiosity, attentiveness, or engagement) or *resistance* (feeling impatience, boredom, sleepiness, or agitation or judging your experience in some way). Mindfulness helps you shift from categorizing an experience into "pleasant" versus "unpleasant" to one of understanding and wisdom through awareness.

As you attune yourself to the breath, not by trying to alter or evaluate the breath in any way but rather by accepting or being with the breath as it is, a tender relationship is developed—you learn to trust and surrender to it. As you do this with the breath, you are better able to be with and trust yourself as well. You uncover places where you get stuck and places where you find calm, becoming more and more of yourself as you learn to let go and open up.

You may worry that mindfulness or meditation will lead to passivity because you are not striving to get anywhere. But mindfulness cultivates qualities that facilitate change and movement. Through a detached-witnessed perspective, you are better able to avoid getting caught in mind traps or unhelpful habits. Ruminations, depressed feelings, and anxious thoughts lose their hold on you. As shared by my MBSR mentor Bob Stahl (Stahl and Goldstein 2010), one of his students said it this way: "Stress used to have me in its grip, now I have stress in my grip and I can let it go."

If you learn to not resist but rather move toward your discomfort, infertility does not necessarily go away, but you start relating to it differently. When you observe what is happening as it unfolds without judging it, it is not the problem you once thought it was. You have "loosened the grip." You are not defective, because infertility does not define who you are. Rather, it is the challenge of fertility that can be met and skillfully worked with. Not only does your relationship to the situation change but you do as well. In the process, even without trying, you are transformed.

ESTABLISHING THE PRACTICE

Meditation is the ship to travel the ocean of the mind. It carries you on the waves, currents, and tides; helps you stay on course; and provides the challenges necessary to cultivate qualities for the journey. The first step in building this vehicle is to set an intention to practice daily. The second step is drawing the plans: when, where, and how to practice. The third step is tracking its course.

Step 1: Set an *intention* to practice ten minutes a day, and consider increasing it to twenty-plus minutes a day. (Instructions for each of the formal practices is described in each chapter, but if you wish to listen to the chapter's guided meditation, go to www.janettimarotta.com/meditations). If you are using the ten-minute guided meditation from my website and you wish to extend your meditation, simply continue on your own. While duration helps to establish depth in your practice, it's consistency that's more important. If you miss a practice, no need for discouragement; just *begin anew.*

Step 2a: Find your *time* to practice. It's hard to sit when already engaged in activity, so practicing soon after you wake up is generally recommended. A morning practice also sets the tone for the whole day. Set your alarm so it rings a bit earlier, and when it goes off, let that be the chime of mindfulness that calls you to the practice. Other recommended times include the transitional times of day, because you're already taking a break from what you were previously doing. These times include returning home from school or work, before lunch, and before bed.

Step 2b: Find your *place* to practice. Create a space for your meditation pillow or chair and place a clock, blanket, and device that plays the guided meditations nearby so you have everything you need at hand. It can be helpful to bring inspirational or calming objects to create a sacred place, such as statues or candles. In time, your heart will be like a magnet and pull you here.

Step 2c: Find your *position*. You can sit cross-legged on the edge of a meditation pillow to protect your lower back from curving and to sustain an upright position, or you can sit on a chair with your feet squarely planted on the floor, without your back resting against the chair so your spine is erect. Close your eyes. Imagine a string on top of your head lifting your upper body toward the sky while your lower body roots to the earth. Place your hands on your thighs—palms up to inspire an attitude of receptivity or palms down to encourage a feeling of stability. Allow the body to "embody" noble qualities, such as nobility, peace, and stability. While meditating, sense states of well-being as they arise, such as peace or calm. This will help draw you to practice. Sit comfortably while maintaining a *relaxed alertness*: a light and gentle *touch* on your object of attention with full awareness. While sitting is the preferred position, lying down or standing up are also options.

Step 3: *Chart* your practice. Use the weekly practice logs at the end of each chapter to help establish or strengthen your mindfulness practice. Just as in meditation, there is no success or failure with how the practice goes each week. If you practiced, what did you learn and how did you benefit? What drew you to practice? What did you learn about the workings of your mind? If you did not practice, what got in the way? What forms did resistance take—too busy, tired, distracted, or wound up? Whatever you notice offers important information about how you get stuck and how you break free from suffering. To help find an effective pattern to your practice, you may also wish to record when and how long you practiced.

Meditation on the Breath

In breath-awareness meditation, you used such supportive tools as counting the breath or marking the breath with touch to help anchor attention. In meditation on the breath, you bring *bare attention* to the breath, coming into intimate contact with the felt sensation of each unfolding breath as it's expressed—*feeling into* the current of the in-breath and out-breath, and noticing how each breath is like a wave, with its own rhythm, movement, texture, tone, and duration without needing to analyze, evaluate, or fix. You also notice how you are *relating to* the breath. Are you relating with resistance (e.g., judgment) or acceptance (e.g., engagement)? When the mind wanders, attention is brought back to breath sensations.

Formal Practice: Meditation on the Breath

For meditation on the breath and the successive practices, make an intention to practice ten minutes or longer each day. Sit on a chair with your feet flat on the floor or on a pillow in a cross-legged position. Settle into an upright, alert yet relaxed posture, with your hands on your lap—palms up in a receptive position or palms down in a grounding position. Notice how the body embodies an attitude—perhaps a feeling of nobility like a king or queen, serenity like a monk or lily floating on a pond, or stability like a mountain or giant sequoia. Feel into this posture, absorbing the quality that radiates from within.

Notice the breath naturally occurring. Gently bring light attention to the breath, noticing breath sensations in the body. You may notice breath sensations in the following:

Belly—ballooning as you breathe in, deflating as you breathe out.

Chest—lifting on the in-breath, lowering on the out-breath.

Whole body—expanding on the inhalation, contracting on the exhalation.

Nostrils—cooling on the entry, warming on the exit.
Upper lip—receding into the nostrils, touching like a breeze as it leaves the nostrils.

Rather than moving attention from one location to another, bring your focus to the area in which the breath is most vivid. As you maintain your focus on the breath, pay close attention to the unique qualities of each breath—texture and tone (smooth or jagged), sensations (flow, rhythm, undulation, rise, fall, lifting, lowering), length and lapse (the out-breath being slightly longer than the in-breath, the moment between the in-breath and out-breath when there is no breath).

As you are sensing and being drawn into the current of the breath in the body, ride the waves of each breath sensation. When the mind wanders, simply make a mental note, "thinking," and then gently shepherd the mind back to the breath, riding on each and every breath sensation. Notice your *relationship* with the breath. Are you relating with resistance (e.g., impatience, boredom, slackening off, lack of interest, sleepiness, agitation, or judgment of your experience in some way) or acceptance (e.g., curiosity, attentiveness, engagement, or at harmony with the breath as it is)?

When ready, end your meditation by congratulating yourself for taking this time for health and healing and slowly open your eyes. Record your meditation on the practice log at the end of the chapter. Note if you related to the breath with resistance, acceptance, or both:

Resistance (feeling impatience, sleepiness, judgment, etc.): Did I impose judgment on myself or my experience as good or bad? Did I lose interest in the breath and find my mind wandering? Did I experience sound as distracting, or did physical discomfort dominate my experience?

Acceptance (feeling curiosity, attentiveness, or engagement): Was I able to "work with" what was actually present—apply neutral attention so I could *turn toward* that which I resist? Was I able to stay with the breath as it is, discovering the unique qualities of each breath? When my mind wandered, did I make a mental note—"thinking"—and then escort my mind back to the breath? Did I bring with me an attitude of curiosity so I could notice patterns of where my mind wandered to, such as planning, worrying, or replaying? Did I sense calm, joy, peace, stability, ease, or other wholesome states arising?

To listen to the guided formal practice of meditation on the breath, go to www.janettimarotta.com/meditations.

The Informal Practice

The informal practice of mindfulness consists of bringing attention to the present moment in everyday life. As you learn to carry mindful awareness into your day, you open to the world of the senses and are able to be more fully present. For example, if you are washing dishes, rather than being distracted with random or judgmental thoughts, such as wishing dishwashing was over so you could get on with the next activity, you simply pay attention to the experience of washing dishes—feeling the sensation of warm water and suds on your hands, noticing how the plate changes from dirty to rinsed off, sensing the movement of the plate as it enters the dishwasher. Through the simple repetitive act of washing dishes that we take for granted (and usually wish we did not need to do), you learn to appreciate and come to know the subtle, dynamic nature of life.

One of the gifts of mindfulness is the ability to pause before reacting. Sometimes referred to as the *wise pause*, informal practices are instrumental in reinforcing this skill. In general, informal practices teach you that by stopping to consciously breathe from the belly, you can disengage from automatic reactivity; observe your thoughts, emotions, and physical sensations; and return to the present moment by bringing awareness back with you (Germer, Siegel, and Fulton 2005, 227).

Informal Practice: Breath Awareness-Pause

Intersperse this two-to-three-minute informal *pause* practice throughout the day. It focuses attention on the breath and is a way to seek refuge from wild thoughts or loose emotions and return to the present moment, where peace and calm reside. Begin by taking two to three deep abdominal breaths. Bring attention to the belly, noticing the rise of the belly on the in-breath and the fall of the belly on the out-breath. Feel the undulation, the rhythm, and the massage of the breath in the body as it signals the body to slow and relax. As you continue to mindfully breathe, expand your awareness to the simple act of what you are doing. If it's walking, feel your feet on the ground as you're taking each step. If it's sitting, notice the contact of the body on the chair, your feet on the floor, and your hands on your lap. If you're washing dishes, experience the feel of the water on your hands and the look of the dishes being rinsed. Bring your full attention to the here and now of whatever activity in which you're engaged.

Create a visual reminder to take a pause. For example, write "pause" on a small object, such as a smooth white pebble, and keep it close at hand—in your pocket or purse or on your desktop or dashboard. Optimal times to take a pause are when you are in a difficult situation, notice feelings of distress, have a natural break, wish to take a break, or need to wait (such as at a stop light, in a waiting room, or in a grocery line). The more you practice taking a pause, the more you naturally choose to pause because it feels like the *wise* thing to do. On the practice log at the end of the chapter, record the cause-effect experience of the pause practice on your everyday life.

Navigating Treatment

Approximately one out of every six couples experiences infertility. Causes of infertility in couples include the following percentages: 35 percent sperm or other male problems, 35 percent problems with the fallopian tubes or uterus, 15 percent problems related to ovulation, and 10–15 percent unexplained causes (Speroff, Glass, and Kase 1999, 1021). Science has made considerable advances, particularly in the last thirty years, to help couples achieve pregnancy through ART. The most significant among these treatments is IVF. Given the best circumstances, many clinics predict a 50 percent IVF pregnancy rate on the first attempt. Successive tries (within three completed attempts) increase the probability of overall success.

Today, even frozen embryo transfers approach the success rate of fresh transfers. Male issues related to poor sperm motility or morphology are treated with a procedure called intracytoplasmic sperm injection (ICSI), which injects a single sperm directly into an egg to enable fertilization. Genetic or miscarriage concerns are addressed with comprehensive chromosomal screening (CCS), in which an embryo biopsy is performed on day five after IVF retrieval to test for genetic abnormalities.

A common mistake is pursuing IVF before it is well understood. Too often, expectations are unrealistic and decisions are made unwisely. "Fertility 101" in the appendix is included to facilitate your understanding of IVF and medical issues surrounding infertility and its treatment.

Because each appointment in the IVF process can lead to unpredictable outcomes and there is a general sense of loss of control, IVF is described as a *roller coaster*. The ramp up for each attempt is slow and deliberate, the falls are fast and sudden, and the twists and turns are jerky and unexpected. At any point, problems can arise: cysts may occur from the initial medication, the uterine lining may not be thick enough, fertilization rate may be poor, or cycles may be canceled before retrieval if there are too few developing follicles. Even though the protocol is precisely followed and financial and emotional resources carefully managed, there is no guarantee of a successful outcome.

The need to obtain a diagnosis, engage in treatment, and deal with potential loss and negative outcomes can be emotionally threatening, and multiple internal and external factors may be involved: denying a problem, feeling low self-worth, believing oneself undeserving, having insufficient funds, waiting to find a marriage partner, remaining overwhelmed with work or life responsibilities, being heavily invested on the career track, having medical problems or family crises—the list goes on.

IVF is a complicated and intensive treatment that gives hope to those pursuing a family, but deciding to take the high-tech route comes with a gamble. IVF can become addictive, and knowing when to stop treatment can be difficult, as there is no way to predict when you are going to *hit the jackpot*. It's hard to say good-bye to a course of treatment that has been so costly in terms of money, time, resources, and energy. But ending treatment can be particularly painful, because it involves letting go of the genetic tie. The question invariably becomes: *when is enough, enough?*

PREPARING FOR IVF

Knowing how to walk the IVF tightrope can only be done by weighing both inner and outer resources with a clear and balanced mind. Mindfulness teaches you how to get out of your own way so you don't get trapped by clinging to what you want as though your life depends on it, avoiding what you don't want even when escape is impossible, or denying the situation by hiding your head in the sand: "what I don't know can't hurt me."

Seeing through the lens of nonjudgmental present-moment awareness enables you to take one step at a time and learn along the way. Each step gives important information about how to take the next. A failed IVF provides data on how to vary the protocol for the next attempt or whether it's worth trying for another round. "A paradox of mindfulness practice is that we never get it right and we never get it wrong" (Germer, Siegel, and Fulton 2005, 114). Every situation is for learning and growth. Even when you are forced to make a decision before you are ready, whatever decision you make is a wholesome decision, *if* you back it up and make it so.

You have financial, emotional, time, and physical bank accounts that need to be managed. When doing so, consider these factors:

- *Financial bank account.* Determining your treatment options and how long you can pursue those options takes money—and lots of it. Plan for the possibilities of failed outcomes so you don't find yourself unable to engage in a result with a high probability of success, such as donor egg IVF. If your medical plan does not have a fertility benefit, consider purchasing fertility insurance.
- *Emotional bank account.* To avoid emotional depletion, it's best to not continuously repeat an option with a high probability of failure. This can drain needed energy to explore other family-building options. If

you know you are inclined to always give your best, you may need to give it "one last try." If you find yourself able to let go and move on, choose among your options.

- *Time bank account.* Factoring in age and how long you've been trying to conceive need serious consideration. It is impossible to know when your fertility challenge will end, but it is possible to know how you can move forward to parenthood. Identify, understand, and consider all options.

- *Physical bank account.* Using hormonal therapy month after month can be physically and emotionally draining. Remember, your holistic prescription for fertility treatment is a balance between medication, procedures, and self-care.

Journal: Overall Bank Account

Take stock of your financial, emotional, time, and physical bank accounts. Are you aware of treatment and parenting options, and do you have the overall capability of pursuing them? In what areas are you depleted or nearly depleted, and what can you do to accumulate more "wealth?" Write a journal entry on your *overall bank account.*

PREPARING FOR INJECTIONS

Visualization is known to effect change in a similar way as the action itself. Visualization is fundamental to some meditation practices and in such diverse arenas as medicine, sports, and music. Runners are trained to imagine being first to cross the finish line; public speakers are coached to envision standing at the podium with a sense of confidence.

Mind-body cancer physician and author Bernie Siegel (1986, 154), tells the story of a young patient with brain cancer who was taught visualization as an adjunct to treatment. When receiving chemotherapy, the little boy imagined the chemicals as rocket ships, as in a video game, flying around in his head shooting at the tumor. Dr. Siegel highlights how this patient's positive relationship with treatment not only enabled him to experience chemotherapy with greater ease, but also potentially increased the effectiveness of his treatment.

Visualization can be used to help deal with many treatment challenges, in particular for IVF-related injections. Especially when there is a fear of needles, this is an aspect of treatment that can be terrifying. Imagining injections as fertile agents can really help.

Exercise: Visualization

When needing to give yourself injections, this visualization exercise helps turn on the relaxation response with abdominal breathing and shifts attention away from the needle and on to visualizing medication as a messenger for fertility.

Begin by taking several long, concentrated breaths—breathing in deeply from your nose and out from your mouth as you expel tension and tightness. Invite the breath to slow and deepen as you start abdominal breathing, noticing your belly expanding on the inhalation and deflating on the exhalation. As you prepare to give yourself the injection, visualize the medication as a fertile agent boosting your body's ability for pregnancy. As the needle enters, imagine hormones balancing, follicles growing, uterine lining building, embryos nestling, or whatever stage of the process hormones are assisting. Give gratitude for these hormones as *potencies of possibility.*

PREPARING FOR THE CALL

My work has been informed over the years by both my clinical practice and my personal infertility experience. When pursuing donor IVF, I tried all sorts of mental tricks to prepare myself for the pregnancy-result call that rings ten long and anxious days after embryo transfer. As for most, this was the hardest part of the treatment cycle. Someone told me the story of an IVF veteran who attempted twenty IVF cycles and offered the following advice: "Have high hopes and low expectations." Though I tried my best to follow this counsel, there was no way to balance such a fine line when the stakes of falling off the tightrope were so high.

Like many attempting fertility treatment, I was advised by friends and family to just *think positive*. If it were only about having positive thoughts! Though well intentioned, most people do not understand how difficult, if not impossible, it is to feel positive when everything up to now has failed or when you are perpetually falling on the unfortunate side of the probability scale.

Consistent with so many women I have worked with, I was afraid to think positive, because if the cycle failed I would feel totally demolished, but I was also afraid to think negative, because if the cycle was unsuccessful it would be my fault. The attempt to feel contrary to how you are actually feeling is a by-product of the coping mechanism of control. Particularly in situations like this, where outcome is not determined by effort, this tactic only increases anxiety and generalized loss of control.

Knowing whether to feel hopeful or hopeless regarding treatment outcomes is another common catch-22. Hope can potentially add to the already turbulent roller-coaster ride of infertility, because it is seeking strength in the future rather than in the present and is paired with perceived success and failure—outcomes over which you have no control. At the same time, entering a cycle with feelings of hopelessness is not productive either. Even though hopeless feelings may protect you from an emotional crash, they put you on track for depression, because each time treatment fails, your emotional baseline starts lower. Because you can only rebound as high as you previously were, you are actually training yourself to be depressed! This is a lesson I and so many women I have worked with have learned to truly take to heart.

If you find yourself juggling between positive and negative thinking or hopeful and hopeless feelings, use your mindfulness meditation training to let attention and intention steer the course.

Bring *attention* to what you can control—the process:

- Follow the treatment protocol as directed. Stay on top of all medical appointments.
- Take care of your physical health—diet, exercise, sleep.

- Attend to your emotional health by practicing mindfulness; accessing support; and engaging in healthy, uplifting activities.
- Engage in the formal and informal mindfulness practices and cultivate such qualities as patience, acceptance, trust, and compassion to guide and support your fertility journey.

Make an *intention* to accept what you cannot control—the outcome:

- Apply mindfulness to your thoughts so you can view the outcome from a neutral perspective. For example:
  ○ "Each IVF provides information on what to do next, bringing me one step closer to having a child."
  ○ "Whatever the outcome, I know I have tried my best and will continue to do so."
  ○ "If IVF is unsuccessful, I know I will have a child if I open to possibilities."

Mindfulness does not imply an unwanted outcome will not bring feelings of sadness or loss or even that you will not emotionally crash or feel depressed. But mindfulness teaches you how to find a place of calm and return to it faster and easier. Even more so, the practice provides the ability to lower stress and cultivate qualities to stay the course of treatment, develop clarity of mind to make wise treatment decisions, choose how you wish to respond to challenging situations, and not take unwanted outcomes as a personal failure.

As you learn to take care of yourself with mindfulness, you are engaging in repeated acts of kindness that become an important part of your fertility journey. Overtime, these recurrent kind deeds become *who* you are.

Exercise: Map

To prepare for the pregnancy result, map out a course of action that will support you through this challenging time. Use this exercise called *MAP*, the acronym for "make a plan."

Thoughts. Are you mindfully framing your thoughts in a way that affirms what you are doing to have a child and how you will still be OK if the cycle fails?

Emotions. What qualities can you cultivate to guide and support your fertility journey, and what can you do to strengthen these attributes?

Actions. Where do you want to get the result (e.g., at home or at work)? Do you want someone to be with you (e.g., your partner)? What will you do afterward (e.g., go to a movie, take a walk)? How will you obtain support (e.g., call a friend, see your counselor)?

Mindful Inquiry: Obstacle Versus Challenge

As you find a comfortable resting position by either lying down on your back or sitting up with a straight spine, slowly close your eyes. Take three deep, long breaths—inhaling through the nostrils, exhaling tension from the mouth. Return to breathing at your own natural rhythm—inhaling and exhaling from your nostrils, inviting the breath to slow and deepen on its own. Ride upon the gentle flow of each breath wave.

When ready, drop into your heart—imagine breathing into and out from your heart. On the inhalation, feel the heart opening and expanding. On the exhalation, feel the heart softening and relaxing. Open to this inquiry practice by asking yourself this question: "Is the obstacle infertility or the challenge fertility?" As your heart opens wide, welcome the answer.

Practice Log 2: Formal Practice--Meditation on the Breath
What did you learn/how did you benefit?   What were your challenges/what interfered?
DAY 1
DAY 2
DAY 3
DAY 4
DAY 5
DAY 6
DAY 7

Practice Log 2: Informal Practice: Breath Awareness - Pause
Note the influence of taking a pause by bringing awareness to the breath.
DAY 1
DAY 2
DAY 3
DAY 4
DAY 5
DAY 6
DAY 7

Three

BEFRIENDING THE BODY

*Realize that this very body, with its aches and its pleasures...is
exactly what we need to be fully human, fully awake, fully alive.*

—PEMA CHODRON

In chapter 3, I introduce you to the foundational practice of mindfulness
of the body. Mindfulness is an *embodied* practice: attention is focused on
how the body responds to thoughts, emotions, and experiences. Mindfulness
teaches that "if the body is relaxed, the mind will follow." When thoughts
weave stories that are often not true and unruly emotions only confirm your
thoughts' worse fears, the body provides trustworthy, direct experience available only in the present moment. Bringing awareness to the body settles, softens, and soothes.

Because you can trust the body as a reliable source of information, when
consciously breathing and placing attention on the body, you become an active
participant in observing the physical manifestations of mental and emotional

stress. Is your heart aching from sadness, head throbbing from anxiety, chest tight from feeling trapped? By inviting the body to relax and let go, you are simultaneously creating distance from disturbing thoughts and loosening the hold of destructive emotions.

Steering toward Discomfort

Kabat-Zinn (1990, 76–79) translated a Buddhist meditation on the body into what he calls "the body scan." This practice systematically sweeps the body with awareness, from the tips of the toes to the crown of the head, identifying sensations in each part of the body, one area at a time. Without judging whether you like or dislike how you're feeling, evaluating the feeling as good or bad, or trying to fix or resist how you're feeling, you *get to know* what each sensation feels like as you delve ever more deeply into the body. When the mind wanders, attention is brought back to the object of attention, in this case body sensations.

Kabat-Zinn describes a kind of intimacy established from the body scan. When you tune in to your body and are mindful of it without judging, "you are reclaiming your own life in that moment and your own body, literally making yourself more real and more alive" (Kabat-Zinn 1990, 76). The compassionate relationship established through a body-awareness practice can be especially potent medicine for fertility challenges, when the body does not feel particularly friendly, forgiving, or welcoming.

Meditation on the Body

Unlike the systematic sweep of the body scan, meditation on the body opens the field of awareness to the body as a whole. Attention moves toward the area of the body where sensations are most vivid and then shifts to the area that draws your attention. Similar to the body scan, you intimately explore and work with sensations with an attitude of nonjudgment. With bare attention, you feel into each region, acknowledging what you're physically feeling in terms of general sensations and the particular quality of each sensation, and you observe how you're relating to sensations—with resistance (e.g., judging, avoiding) or acceptance (e.g., being with sensations as they are). You learn to use the breath to make room for sensations to soften, soothe, or simply be. When the mind wanders, attention is brought back to body sensations.

The very act of acknowledging what you're feeling is a powerful mechanism of discharging tension, as it's your resistance to pain or discomfort that intensifies pain. By turning toward discomfort rather than fighting against it, sensations soften on their own. As you learn how to be with discomfort, you're cultivating the quality of "letting be"—accepting things as they are, without grasping onto them or pushing them away. Meditation on the body prepares you for the succeeding practices, which teaches how to work with mental turmoil and emotional distress.

Formal Practice: Meditation on the Body

To practice meditation on the body, lie on your back or sit upright with your eyes closed. Gently tune in to breath sensations in the body and ride upon the ebb and flow of the in-breath and out-breath.

Open your awareness now to the sense of touch. Feel how every place on your body is touched by the mat or chair, floor, clothes, and air. As you're cradled in the blanket of touch, expand your awareness to notice skin sensations and internal sensations throughout the body (muscles and connective tissue, veins, arteries, and blood flow, organs and bones). You may notice temperature variation (hot, cold, warm, cool), density (tightness, tension, numbness), movement (tingling, trembling, shaking), and neutralness (which is also a feeling). Direct your attention to wherever sensation becomes most noticeable, vibrant, or active.

As you acknowledge sensations, allow them to be as they are without trying to get rid of them or cling to them. Breathe into and out from sensations, making room for sensations to soften, dissipate, or simply be, or just invite the breath to ride the waves of any sensation. When the mind wanders, bring the mind back to the object of attention, in this case body sensation.

Notice if you are relating to body sensations with resistance (e.g., judgment, irritation) or acceptance (e.g., being with sensations as they are). Return to the breath to calm and stabilize if the sensation is too intense or difficult to stay with.

When ready, end with two to three full-body-cleansing breaths: on the in-breath, scan the body for any remaining tension from the base of your feet up your legs, spine, neck, and head; on the out-breath, blow any remaining dust and debris from the imaginary "blowhole" on top of your head. Return to natural breathing, sensing the body as a whole. When ready, slowly open your eyes.

On the practice log at the end of the chapter, record what you learned and how you benefitted. If you didn't practice, what were your challenges and what interfered? Remember, there is no success, no failure. Everything is here for the learning! To listen to the guided meditation that complements this chapter's formal practice, go to www.janettimarotta.com/meditations.

Informal Practice: Body Awareness-Pause

This two-to-three-minute informal pause practice can be used in a tense situation or at any time throughout the day. It focuses attention on the body as a way to stop the mind's obsessive chatter and to extinguish fuming emotions.

Begin by taking two to three deep abdominal breaths. Return to natural breathing and observe the following:

Thoughts—what are you thinking? Without trying to interpret or analyze, simply acknowledge your dominant thought (e.g., "I know the doctor will give me bad news").

Emotions—what are you feeling emotionally? Without clinging to your feelings, trying to avoid them, or identifying with them, simply acknowledge and label your dominant emotion (e.g., if it's anxiety, say to yourself, "This is anxiety").

Body Sensations—what are you feeling physically? Focus most of your time here, noticing points of tension and, through breath and movement, inviting the body to release and unwind. For example, if you sense

- tension in your jaw—open your mouth wide and close it two or three times.
- stiffness in the neck—circle your head in one direction a few times and then in the other direction a few times.
- fidgety hands and fingers—massage your hands, one finger at a time.
- an aching heart—imagine breathing from your heart: on the in-breath, visualize the heart expanding, and on the out-breath, visualize the heart softening.
- tight muscles—imagine breathing into and out from places of tension, giving room for sensations to run their course or be as they are.
- tension in the whole body—stretch, bend, twist, wiggle, shake, or massage.

To end, make an intention to bring this calm, centered, awake attention with you. Use a visual reminder to strengthen the practice; for example, write "pause" on a white pebble, glass bead, or eraser and keep it close at hand. Remember, the more you practice taking a pause, the more you will naturally choose to pause, because it feels like the *wise* thing to do.

On the practice log at the end of the chapter, record the cause-effect experience of the pause practice. How did you benefit from this practice?

Finding Your Edge through Yoga

Yoga, the Sanskrit word for "to integrate," brings the mind and body into balance and as such is a kind of meditation. Yoga uses postures to show your *edge*—that place of balance where you're not overdoing or underdoing. In particular, the practice cultivates the quality of nonstriving—not trying to get anywhere except into the present moment. As you learn to stretch and balance with *right effort*, or alert and relaxed attention, you are learning how to work with mental and emotional turmoil and how to bring this ability to your experience throughout the day. Yoga serves as a practice ground for daily living, opening a doorway to freedom from suffering.

The practice teaches how to work with physical discomfort and utilizes the breath to soften places of tightness. Yoga teaches that the breath wields a potent effect on the body and mind. As you work with postures, you notice that when the breath is shallow, rapid, or held, physical and emotional tension increases, but when the breath is slow, long, and steady, postures can be sustained longer, stretching extends further, and there's a sense of greater ease.

As a mindfulness practice, you maintain awareness on the present moment by aiming your attention on the posture and your intention on sustaining the posture. When attention wanders, you make a mental note (e.g., "thinking") and then gently return to the posture. While in the posture, awareness is directed to body sensations, breathing space into and out from regions of greatest intensity. As you ride the waves of your breathing, you relax and sink into each posture.

Mindful Yoga for Fertility

Why is yoga part of a mindfulness approach to fertility? Yoga reestablishes a welcoming connection to the body. Yoga nourishes and strengthens the parasympathetic nervous system, reinforcing the relaxation response. When movement is added to the breath, stress and bodily tension diminish. Circulation, blood flow, and energy in the reproductive organs increase. Oxygen to the central nervous system is raised, abdominal organs are toned and massaged, and overall energy is fostered.

Hatha yoga is the recommended yoga for fertility and combines physical exercises (asanas) and breathing techniques (pranayama) to stimulate the glandular system and increase vital energy. The most popular styles of yoga taught in Western culture today are all forms of hatha yoga. While mindful awareness is naturally embedded into yoga, some yoga teachers accentuate mindfulness into the practice more than others.

Specific styles of yoga suggested for fertility include restorative yoga, which uses props to support postures and encourage gentle release, and yin yoga, which focuses on female energy. Bikram, ashtanga, and power yoga are not recommended for fertility, particularly bikram yoga, which is practiced in a heated room, because of its overheating, overworking effect on the body.

When on stimulating hormones during a treatment cycle, it's critical to avoid twisting movements, such as flip turns while swimming or high-impact exercise like jogging. Ovaries can torque or turn upside down because they are heavier and enlarged, resulting in loss of a functioning ovary. To be on the cautious side, avoid practicing yoga during this period.

Though not validated by Western research, some yoga teachers believe there are postures to avoid and others that are conducive for fertility. Unfavorable yoga postures include those that put pressure on the pelvic area or lower back, including back bends and Cobra pose, or intense inversions, such as headstands. Beneficial yoga poses (which are all described in the yoga sequence) include the following: Downward-Facing Dog and Yawning Cat, which strengthen and lengthen the spine, increase energy, and stimulate glands; Forward-Folding Bend, which activates the hypothalamus-pituitary-adrenal axis to potentially help balance hormones; Bridge pose, which activates the thyroid (critical for fertility); and Sitting Twist, which massages abdominal organs, releases toxins, and stimulates digestion. Lying on your back with your legs at a ninety-degree angle up against the wall is considered to be especially helpful to increase reproductive circulation.

For all types of yoga, these general breathing principles apply:

Breathe out with any movement that contracts your belly and front side of your body, when bending down from waist, while lifting one leg when lying on your back.

Breathe in with any movement that expands the front side of your body and contracts your backside, when bending up from your waist, while lifting one leg while lying on your belly.

Slowly ease into poses, knowing that over time flexibility increases. For example, begin Downward-Facing Dog with knees bent and heels off the mat. Gradually you will be able to straighten your legs and release your heels to the mat. Know that if any of the poses are held too long, you can always come out of them. Take a break in Yawning Cat, which is especially restorative. Always check with your doctor or physical therapist if you have a physical condition that can be exacerbated by a posture.

Formal Practice: Mindful Yoga For Fertility

This mindful yoga for fertility practice consists of a fourteen-posture sequence. Because this week introduces you to two formal practices, you may wish to alternate the meditation in stillness practice (meditation on the body) with this meditation in movement practice (mindful yoga for fertility). When following the guided yoga practice on www.janettimarotta.com/meditations, the postures are divided into two ten-minute practices which you can do separately or back-to-back. Use the practice chart at the end of this chapter to record your practice.

To prepare for yoga, place a mat on the floor to establish your personal practice space and have a pillow or blanket available. Wear clothing that allows for easy stretching and remove your socks so your feet have traction on the mat.

1. Sitting Pose

- Place your folded blanket or pillow on your mat. Sit cross-legged on the edge of it with your knees toward the floor, taking the sway out of your lower back and placing it in a neutral position.

- Sit with a straight back and elongated spine, with your shoulders down and relaxed, head square with your shoulders, and chin slightly in.
- Place your hands with palms up on your knees.
- Close your eyes as you feel into this pose. Notice the felt sensations of this posture and how this posture embodies an attitude or quality of stability, calmness, or balance. Tune in to the natural rhythm of your breath. As you ride on the current of the breath waves in the body, bring into your heart the deep motivation for being here, recognizing this practice is an act of love.

2. ARMS WIDE LIKE A BIRD

- From Sitting pose, place your hands to your sides with palms up. Take a long deep inhalation—raising arms wide like a bird, fingers splayed, feeling the opposing arm extension—sensing where you are in movement.
- When your palms touch as you reach toward the sky, take a long, deep exhalation—lowering arms wide like a bird, fingers splayed, feeling the opposing arm extension—sensing where you are in movement.
- With your arms to your sides, for several natural breaths, sense where you are in stillness.
- Repeat.

3. SHOULDER AND NECK STRETCH

- On the inhalation, bring your shoulders to your ears, holding them there as you feel the tension. On the exhalation, let them drop as you feel the release. Repeat.
- As you breathe with awareness at your own pace, bring your shoulders forward and then backward. Repeat. Bring your left ear toward the left shoulder, without lifting up your shoulder, and then your right ear toward the right shoulder, without lifting up your shoulder. Repeat.

Bring your head forward and then backward. Repeat. Turn your head in small, then larger, gentle circles in one direction and then the other direction. Repeat.

- Shake out your shoulders, moving them vigorously in any direction, releasing remaining tension.

4. COBBLER'S POSE

- Bring the soles of your feet together toward the center of your body, bending your knees out to form a diamond shape.
- Hold on to your feet and move toward the center of your body, or place your hands behind your back and move the center of your body toward your feet.
- Relax your shoulders and elongate your neck with chin in, allowing knees to open as you're sitting tall. Breathe with awareness as you're releasing into the pose.

5. SITTING TWIST

- Return to Sitting pose with your legs crossed, knees toward the floor with a straight back and elongated spine.
- On the inhalation, stretch your arms over your head like a bird. On the exhalation, turn to the right with your right hand on the floor as far as the twist permits, placing your left hand on the side of your right hip. Breathe with awareness into this twist. Notice how you can stretch farther on the out-breath—on the "letting go" breath. When ready, come back to neutral.
- Reverse. On the inhalation, stretch your arms over your head like a bird. On the exhalation, turn to the left with your left hand on the floor as far as the twist permits, placing your right hand on the side of your left hip. Breathe with awareness into this twist. Notice the stretch increase with the out-breath—the "letting go" breath. When ready, come back to neutral.
- Feel the breath in the body as you feel into the benefits of this twisting stretch.

6. Cat-Cow

- From Sitting pose, place your hands and knees on the mat with a flat tabletop back.
- On the inhalation, raise your head and tailbone up as the belly lowers (sagging cow). Consciously breathe for several breaths into this pose. Reverse. On the exhalation, drop your head and tailbone as the back curves up (Halloween cat). Consciously breathe for several breaths into this pose.
- For several stretches now, coordinate each move with the rhythm of the breath—inhaling into sagging cow, exhaling into Halloween cat.
- Return to tabletop position as you breathe with awareness and feel into the consequences of this spinal stretch and release.

7. Downward-Facing Dog

- With your hands flat on the mat, fingers splayed, and arms slightly bent, raise your buttocks up, moving your body into the shape of a triangle as you place your feet on the mat with heels stretched toward the floor as far as comfortable. Relax the legs with knees ideally straight (if possible), being careful not to overdo this stretch.
- Relax your shoulders away from the ears, elongating the body between your hands and feet by moving your raised hips back. Relax your head with your neck down and chin in. Hold this position for several conscious breaths as you feel into this stretch.

8. Yawning Cat

- From Downward-Facing Dog, bend your knees, dropping your buttocks toward the heels with the top of your feet on the mat.
- Stretch your arms out in front of you, with palms down, fingers splayed, and forehead resting on the mat.
- For several conscious breaths, rest in the relaxing effects of this pose.

9. DOWNWARD-FACING DOG

- From Yawning Cat pose, return to Downward-Facing Dog with your hands flat on the floor, buttocks up, and feet on the mat with heels stretched toward the floor into a triangle shape position.
- Hold this position again as you feel into this stretch while you breathe deeply and consciously.

10. FORWARD-FOLDING BEND

- From Downward-Facing Dog, on the exhalation walk both feet between your hands. Breathe into this pose with knees bent, gradually straightening legs if possible.
- On the inhalation, lift up from your hips one vertebrae at a time, arms hanging to the side, with your head being last to uncurl.

11. MOUNTAIN POSE

- As you stand upright in Mountain pose, with your feet slightly apart and weight evenly distributed on hips, close your eyes. Have your knees slightly bent, chest open, palms open, head balanced between the shoulders, chin parallel to floor, shoulders released, and back of pelvis straight.
- Breathe long, deep breaths as you stand firm and upright as a mountain—solid, stable, and secure.

12. BRIDGE

- Move into a lying-down position on your back, with arms at your sides and knees bent.

- On the inhalation, lift your buttocks and lower back off the mat, belly toward the sky and chin relaxed. On the exhalation, lower down one vertebrae at a time to the mat.
- Repeat a few more times at your own pace, coordinating the in-breath and out-breath with each opposing move.

13. HUGGING KNEES

- From Bridge pose, move into this counter pose as you hug your knees and move in different directions—rolling side to side and forward to backward with your head on and off the mat—consciously breathing throughout.
- When ready, lower your knees to lie flat on the mat.

14. OPENNESS POSE

- As you're lying on the mat with your eyes closed, open your legs with arms to the side, palms toward the sky. Relax your shoulders, feeling your hips wide and heavy.
- Soften your breath in the belly, inviting your eyes to relax, jaw to let loose, and tongue to release. Invite your body to relax and sink into the earth, allowing the benefits of the practice to soak in.
- As you rest in this pose, feel the vulnerability and immense courage that arise from this position of openness. Congratulate yourself for taking this time for healing and renewal.

Practice Log 3: Formal Practice—Meditation on the Body Mindful Yoga for Fertility
What did you learn/how did you benefit? What were your challenges/what interfered?
DAY 1
DAY 2
DAY 3
DAY 4
DAY 5
DAY 6
DAY 7

Practice Log 3: Informal Practice—Body Awareness - Pause

Note the influence of taking a pause by bringing awareness to the body.

DAY 1

DAY 2

DAY 3

DAY 4

DAY 5

DAY 6

DAY 7

Four

Rejuvenating Holistically

*It is good to have an end to journey toward; but
it is the journey that matters, in the end.*

—Ursula Le Guin

In this chapter, we explore the relationship between self-care and fertility. Developing a mindful, fertile lifestyle can bring a sense of intentionality to the loss of control that permeates infertility. Mindfully choosing what you eat; how you tend the body through exercise, rest, and stress reduction; and whether to add alternative approaches not only optimizes health and well-being but may boost fertility as well.

Based on figures from the National Center for Health Statistics, Center for Disease Control, and National Institutes of Health, America is experiencing a health crisis. Today's population places the responsibility on the medical-care system rather than on our own selves. Only 10 percent of medical care contributes to health-care outcome, while 50 percent of health status is a result of lifestyle choices. Heredity and environment are each reported to contribute 20 percent.

The tendency to focus on pharmaceuticals and procedures in exchange for self-help measures is not only found in general medicine today but in the area of fertility as well:

> While millions upon millions of dollars have been spent developing and perfecting reproductive technologies, almost no attention has been paid to connections between diet and fertility. This oversight speaks volumes to the role of medicine in America—a laser-like focus on drugs, devices, or procedures, that can generate revenue and often total disregard for self-help measures that anyone can do for free. (Chavarro, Willett, and Skerrett 2008, 2)

Though ART increases your probability of success for many fertility issues, it is certainly less than 100 percent. Because of its cost, amount of time required, invasiveness of procedures, and side effects, it is not an option for everyone. Becoming an active participant in your medical care is not only free but freeing.

Journey, Not Destination

I have often seen women putting the "cart before the horse"—trying to get pregnant with medication, surgeries, and procedures without taking care of themselves. Alcoholics Anonymous (AA) is a program founded on the principle of self-care, emphasizing the need to put recovery first, as everything follows from there. When the horse is in front of the cart, the cart just naturally trails behind. While AA advocates "one day at a time," mindfulness puts it this way: "one moment at a time." Contained within each *mind moment* is the invitation to take care of your mental, emotional, and physical well-being. Focus is on the process (how you're actively caring for yourself) rather than on the goal (where you lose yourself and have no control).

Boosting Fertility

In their groundbreaking book *The Fertility Diet* (2008), researchers Chavarro, Willett, and Skerrett examine the role of diet, exercise, and weight control on fertility. Their well-known Nurses' Health Study followed more than eighteen thousand women trying to get pregnant over an eight-year period. Its focus was on ovulatory infertility or problems related to the maturation or release of a mature egg each month (not infertility due to physical impediments such as blocked fallopian tubes), and it gave recommendations for prevention and reversal of ovulatory infertility.

DIET

Overall, the Nurses' Health Study underscores the value of a healthy, well-balanced diet, rich in fruits, vegetables, and whole grains, similar to how we naturally ate before food became processed and refined. Their suggestions bring food "back to basics."

Recommendations and bases for recommendations include the following:

- Slow carbohydrates (whole grains, beans, vegetables, whole fruits), not fast carbs (white rice, potatoes, cold cereal).
  - Slowly digested carbs rich in fiber keep blood sugar and insulin levels low; high levels disrupt the finely tuned balance of hormones needed for reproduction or ovulation. It is not so much the amount of carbs but the quality of carbs that affects fertility. Rapidly digested carbs raise blood sugar and insulin levels that decrease fertility.
- Only monounsaturated fats, no trans fats (stick margarine, French fries, doughnuts).

- ○ Artificial trans fats in fast, baked, and processed foods significantly dampen ovulation and conception. Fats are building blocks for hormones and turn genes on or off, calming inflammation and affecting cell function. Unsaturated fats improve fertility by increasing insulin sensitivity and cooling inflammation.
- More protein from plants and less from animals.
  - ○ More protein from plants and less from animals, which contain different proteins, improves ovulatory infertility, which may influence blood sugar, sensitivity to insulin, and the production of insulin-like growth factor 1.
- Whole milk, not skim or reduced fat. This includes one to two servings of whole milk and foods from whole milk (full fat yogurt, cottage cheese, ice cream).
  - ○ Whole milk is fertility enhancing because removing fat from milk changes its balance of sex hormones necessary for fertility. Proteins added to make skim and low-fat milk further affect the delicate hormonal balance.

The Nurses' Diet does not give specific recommendations on organic food. Keep in mind that eating organic, when possible, decreases exposure to pesticide residue and growth hormones. Organic foods worth considering include milk, beef, and poultry. The Environmental Working Group identifies the "Dirty Dozen," produce that offers the highest pesticide residue, and the "Clean Fifteen," produce with the lowest pesticide residue. For easy reference, you can download a copy of the 2017 wallet guide for the "Dirty Dozen" and "Clean Fifteen" from www.ewg.org/foodnews/.

The Dirty Dozen	The Clean Fifteen
Strawberries	Sweet corn
Spinach	Avocado
Nectarines	Pineapple
Apples	Cabbage
Peaches	Onions
Pears	Sweet peas
Cherries	Papayas
Grapes	Asparagus
Celery	Mangos
Tomatoes	Eggplant
Sweet bell peppers	Honeydew melon
Potatoes	Kiwi
	Cantaloupe
	Cauliflower
	Grapefruit

Some health practitioners recommend eating dark chocolate in moderation because it's an antioxidant—and also a great indulgent. All practitioners caution against overeating soy, because it mimics estrogen.

Increased attention to fertility-enhancing food is definitely on the rise, but recommended foods can change like fads and add increased stress. I have seen many women feel guilty about what they're eating, deprived by food restrictions, or confused by conflicting recommendations. What are you to do? Listen to yourself. Follow the advice of the health-care provider to whom you feel most aligned or the recommendations that feel most right for you.

BODY WEIGHT

Findings from the Nurse's Health Study and other research support a weight zone on the body mass index (BMI) that optimizes fertility, called the "fertile zone." Studies have found ovulation problems and increased risk of miscarriage is often related to being overweight or underweight. Excess weight appears to lower IVF success rate; increase risk during pregnancy of preeclampsia, diabetes, and need for cesarean section; and have effects on the baby. Being ten pounds underweight results in more of a problem than being ten pounds overweight, as the body needs a certain amount of fat to reproduce.

Chavarro, Willett, and Skerrett suggest preliminary studies on men indicate overweight men are less fertile, as excess weight can lower testosterone levels, destabilize the testosterone-estrogen ratio, and dampen sperm motility. Though a fertile zone for men has not yet been established, keeping weight down may be important for increased fertility and is certainly important for overall health.

FERTILE ZONE

Below is a table to determine your body mass index (BMI) and see if you fall within the "fertile zone" (Google Images). To use the table, find your height in the left-hand column, and then move across the row to find your weight. The number at the top of the column is the BMI for that height and weight. BMIs between 19 and 24 lie within the *fertile zone*. Under 19 is considered underweight, 25–29 overweight and 30–35 obese.

Underweight <18.5 Normal 18.5 - 24.9 Overweight 25.0 - 29.0 Obese 30.0 - 34.9

BMI	19	20	21	22	23	24	25	26	27	28	29	30	35	40
Height (in.)	Weight (lb.)													
	-----------------normal---------------							----------overweight----------				------obese------			
58	91	96	100	105	110	115	119	124	129	134	138	143	167	191
59	94	99	104	109	114	119	124	128	133	138	143	148	173	198
60	97	102	107	112	118	123	128	133	138	143	148	153	179	204
61	100	106	111	116	122	127	132	137	143	148	153	158	185	211
62	104	109	115	120	126	131	136	142	147	153	158	164	191	218
63	107	113	118	124	130	135	141	146	152	158	163	169	197	225
64	110	116	122	128	134	140	145	151	157	163	169	174	204	232
65	114	120	126	132	138	144	150	156	162	168	174	180	210	240
66	118	124	130	136	142	148	155	161	167	173	179	186	216	247
67	121	127	134	140	146	153	159	166	172	178	185	191	223	255
68	125	131	138	144	151	158	164	171	177	184	190	197	230	262
69	128	135	142	149	155	162	169	176	182	189	196	203	236	270
70	132	139	146	153	160	167	174	181	188	195	202	207	243	278
71	136	143	150	157	165	172	179	186	193	200	208	215	250	286
72	140	147	154	162	169	177	184	191	199	206	213	221	258	294
73	144	151	159	166	174	182	189	197	204	212	219	227	265	302
74	148	155	163	171	179	186	194	202	210	218	225	233	272	311
75	152	160	168	176	184	192	200	208	216	224	232	240	279	319
76	156	164	172	180	189	197	205	213	221	230	238	246	287	328

PHYSICAL EXERCISE

The Nurses' Health Study highlights the importance of exercise and shows a vital link between activity and becoming pregnant. It explains how muscles need a constant push and pull to stay healthy, respond to insulin effectively, and absorb blood sugar efficiently and how inactivity can lead to excess blood sugar and insulin in the bloodstream, which compromises ovulation, conception, and pregnancy.

The Nurses' Health Study recommends exercising in moderation thirty minutes a day, adjusting exercise by aiming for the fertility zone, without overdoing or underdoing. Exercising regularly also helps to keep your body fit enough to carry pregnancy with ease. All studies advise against prolonged exercise, as it is known to decrease fertility. This is dramatically demonstrated in marathon runners who stop menstruating. While Chavarro, Willett, and Skerrett are not able to offer a specific prescription, they point to four categories of helpful exercise: aerobic exercise, strength training, stretching, and activities of daily living. These activities not only keep muscles healthy and blood sugar and insulin down but also serve as natural stress relievers.

The Nurses' Health Study takes an evolutionary perspective to support the role of exercise on fertility. It points to the activity level of our ancestors—hunting for game, scavenging for food, preparing fields for harvest, and traveling nomadically—burning two times the calories as today's average American.

The effect of exercise for men has more to do with the need for sperm to be kept cooler than normal body temperature. While normal body temperature is 98.6 degrees, normal temperature for testicles is 98 degrees. Sperm is kept cooler because testicles are separated from the body. To enhance sperm production, it is recommended to avoid taking hot tubs, stop wearing tight underwear, and limit jogging and biking.

While exercise is important for women, please remember to avoid high-impact exercise and twisting movements when taking fertility-enhancing drugs during treatment cycles, as this can torque the ovaries. After IVF retrieval, it is recommended to go home and relax, as retrievals are surgical procedures and involve the use of anesthesia. After transfer, it is recommended to take it easy for a day or two and then resume normal activities, with the exception of heavy lifting. Always seek aftercare advice from your fertility physician.

CAFFEINE

Caffeine has been found to potentially increase the rate of miscarriage and lower pregnancy rates. Prior to attempting to conceive and while pregnant, it is generally advised to drink small amounts of caffeine (e.g., one cup of non-strong coffee a day). Remember caffeine is also found in tea (particularly black tea), chocolate, and some soda and energy drinks.

NICOTINE

Smoking has been found to reduce sperm count and motility in men and significantly impact fertility and reduce IVF success rate in women. Smoking changes cervical mucus in women and can constrict blood flow to the placenta, resulting in low birth weight. It is strongly recommended to quit smoking before attempting pregnancy and while pregnant (www.pamf.org/fertility).

ALCOHOL AND DRUGS

Research suggests alcohol and marijuana reduce sperm count in men. Women who consume an excess or moderate amount of alcohol during pregnancy have babies born with fetal alcohol syndrome (FAS), characterized by mental retardation and cranial facial deformities. Alcohol decreases fertility in some women and can add time to becoming pregnant. The use of drugs during pregnancy adversely affects the fetus, with some drugs causing babies to be born addicted. For these reasons, and for overall general health, drug use and alcohol consumption is to be avoided.

ENVIRONMENTAL TOXIN EXPOSURES

Research on the effects of toxic substances on fertility recommends minimized exposure to radioactive materials, industrial solvents, pesticides, and insecticides. Due to the presence of a parasite infection called toxoplasmosis, avoid handling litter boxes. Wash hands, utensils, and cutting boards after handling raw meat (www.pamf.org/fertility).

ACUPUNCTURE

Acupuncture has now become popular in the United States for many diagnoses, including infertility. Robin Sheared, LAC, clinical director of Blue Ova Health (www.blueova.com), described for me why acupuncture is helpful for fertility:

> Acupuncture has a long history of optimizing fertility and supporting conception by improving egg and sperm quality, thus increasing pregnancy and live birth rates. In our clinic, when we see patients twice a week for a minimum of 12 weeks, we can double the live birth rate for women trying to conceive naturally or with IUI/IVF. Similar results are backed up by numerous clinical studies performed over the last decade (Hullender Rubin et al. 2015). Acupuncture before and after ART (assisted reproductive technology such as IUI and IVF) improves egg quality and increases blood flow to the uterus and ovaries (Paulus et al. 2002). Combining acupuncture with western fertility treatments also increases implantation rates during embryo transfer by encouraging an optimal uterine lining. Acupuncture can also reduce stress and anxiety associated with infertility, helping to prevent miscarriage and early pregnancy loss, as well as decreasing side effects from the ART medications. Acupuncture is also extremely effective in improving sperm parameters in terms of count, morphology and motility (Pei et al. 2005). In our clinic, we expect to see notable increases and improvement in sperm when treating our male patients for 12 weeks.

HERBAL REMEDIES

Most acupuncturists include herbs as an important treatment component. Ingredients in herbs are not tightly controlled, and mixing fertility drugs with herbs creates interactive effects. Consult your physician before integrating herbs into your assisted-reproduction treatment protocol.

VITAMINS

It is recommended to take a multivitamin containing folic acid when trying to get pregnant. Research suggests folic acid reduces the risk of such birth defects as spinal bifida, cleft lip, and neural tubal defects (www.pamf.org/fertility). Some fertility specialists advise men to add zinc, which is important for production of normal, healthy sperm.

STRESS REDUCTION

Even the best fertility plan is compromised if stress reduction is not included. Stress promotes short-term solutions, failure to take action, and feelings of powerlessness, which displace responsibility on the medical-care system. Stress reduction enables you to become an active participant in your medical care and make healthy lifestyle choices. As previously noted, studies have determined stress is the number-one reason for dropping out of fertility treatment, and stress reduction in the form of psychosocial interventions has been found to double pregnancy rates. While it's important to make medical appointments, don't forget to book time for yourself!

Exercise: Fertile Lifestyle Plan

What changes would you like to aspire toward to optimize your fertile health and overall wellness? Check the following lifestyle behaviors if they apply, and then consider the corresponding recommendations to develop your own personal plan. It's always a good idea to seek advice from your physician.

_____*Weight/BMI*—My weight is above or below the optimal fertile zone.

To lose or gain weight, bring mindful awareness into when, why, and what you eat. Taking the "wise pause" creates the ability to shift from emotional eating to conscious eating, where healthy food choices can be made.

_____*Diet*—I do not have a balanced diet.

Balance your diet with fruits, vegetables, and whole grains. Consider eating organic foods.

_____*Nicotine*—I smoke cigarettes.

Eliminate all smoking by enrolling in a program or utilizing treatment strategies.

_____*Alcohol*—I drink more than five alcoholic beverages a week.

Reduce consumption. If you believe alcohol is a problem, seek treatment.

_____*Caffeine*—I drink more than one cup of coffee a day.

Reduce caffeine by cutting down a half cup per week to avoid withdrawal.

_____*Marijuana*—I smoke marijuana.

Eliminate marijuana. If you believe marijuana is a problem, seek treatment.

_____*Nutritional supplements*—I am not taking nutritional supplements.

Add nutritional supplements—men may want to consider Fertility Blend.

_____*Acupuncture and traditional Chinese medicine*—I am not in treatment with an acupuncturist.

Consider the option of adding acupuncture to your treatment protocol.

_____*Exercise*—I exercise more than a moderate amount or not at all.

Engage in moderately aerobic activity, such as yoga, chi kung, Pilates, walking, or swimming.

_____*Self-care*—My life is out of balance, and I do not prioritize self-care.

Balance your life with work and play and give precedence to taking care of yourself.

_____*Stress*—I feel depressed, anxious, or isolated.

Develop a mindfulness practice as a "way of being." Pursue counseling or participating in a self-help or group-led fertility mindfulness program.

Mindful Eating

In large part, our national health crisis has to do with what is now recognized as an "epidemic of stress." Depression and stress fuel obesity, which has become a health issue of epic concern. Our brain is wired to seek dense calories in times of stress. It has been determined that sugar consumption has tripled in the last twenty years and that sugar causes addiction.

Stress activates cortisol, which stimulates the brain to seek high-fat, sweet food. What comes out of the ground is fat and sugar, but not both combined. Along with today's overexposure to highly caloric food, it's this fat-sugar combo that stimulates the reward center in the brain to become addicted. Don't be fooled—this same reward phenomenon occurs with diet sweeteners as well.

We're caught in an endless stream of craving, and the neutral lens of mindfulness enables you to look into the nature of craving. Mindfulness teaches that clinging to what you want or don't want is at the root of suffering. This is why overeating and excessive restraint triggers addiction. Mindfulness elucidates the impermanent nature of all things—that craving and pleasure doesn't last. When longing for a particular food or drink, notice how tightly you are holding on to the need for pleasure and try loosening the grip. If all mindfulness practices are reduced to one thing, it's the practice of *letting go*.

Buddhist psychology recommends the "Middle Path." While eating, make an intention to not overeat or undereat, but to eat in moderation. As an embodied practice, mindfulness is an effective way to lose weight. When listening to your body, you start making connections to the consequences of food choices. You hear your body say it's full, this drink is too sweet, or that food is too salty.

Connecting to the cause-effect relationship between craving and contentment generalizes to all areas of life. The insight developed from mindfulness helps end desire, because you are able to look into the true nature of experience and your real needs. As you learn to experience contentment without fulfilling your desire, wisdom develops.

When going to the grocery store, it's never advised to go shopping on an empty stomach, as this increases impulse buying. Plan in advance what you want to eat and go shopping with a list in hand. Notice how much easier it is to make healthy food choices.

When feeling compelled to eat a particular food that may not be your healthiest choice, take the wise pause. Observe whether your desire to eat is being driven by emotional eating—when you're eating to satisfy an emotional need. If so, look at your options. Perhaps you need to step back from what you're doing and soothe yourself in some way, such as a brief meditation, yoga stretch, or walk outside. Proceed with a healthy choice.

MBSR uses what's called the "raisin exercise" (Kabat-Zinn 1990, 27–28) to develop appreciation of each moment by bringing awareness to even the most mundane activity. In this exercise, you eat a raisin with a beginner's mind—looking at things as if it's the first time, without assumptions.

Very slowly and mindfully, you systematically explore the sensations of sight, smell, sound, and taste and describe what you notice. Without interpreting what you notice (what it reminds you of), you simply identify the raisin's qualities—for example, for the sense of sight you might notice brown, ridges, or glistening. If your mind wanders into judgment (e.g., "This is a really dumb exercise"), you simply make a mental note—"judgment"—and return to experiencing the raisin one sense at a time.

Everyone's experience is somewhat different, not better or worse. Quite commonly, participants are surprised by how much more they appreciate the taste of the raisin. Occasionally, participants will notice why they really don't like raisins at all. I captured my experience with the raisin exercise in the following poem:

Raisin'
I called you Raisin.
Brown, sweet, squishy.
Comes in a little red box I can hold in my hand.
But now that I've looked at you,
I see your glistening, dark, amber hues

with crevices and scales.
Now that I've smelled you,
I inhale your pungent fragrance.
I hear your clicks and snaps
when I listen to you move.
As my fingers feel your squish and squirm
and my tongue tastes your tang and tart,
you're raisin' my belly with the inhale
and raisin' awareness with the exhale.

In the book *Peace is Every Step* (1992, 21–22), Thich Nhat Hanh encourages students to look deeply into experience. One of the many practices in this wonderful little book is an eating-awareness exercise that involves an orange. While consciously breathing and having an attitude of a beginner's mind, he suggests holding an orange in your hand, slowly peeling it, smelling its scent, and breaking off one piece at a time to taste it fully. Nhat Hanh explains that as you look at the life history of the orange—the sun and rain on the tree, the blossoms sprouting, and the tiny green fruit emerging and then turning yellow as it grows bigger and bright orange as it fully matures—you see the world in the orange and yourself as part of the world. Nhat Hanh teaches when you are present for the orange, the orange is here for you. The realization emerges that this orange, or any fruit, is "nothing less than a miracle."

Informal Practice: Mindful Eating

For one meal or snack each day this week, practice mindful eating. Engage all your senses by slowing down: *see* the food, noticing texture, shape, size, and color; *smell* the food and inhale the aromas; *hear* the food as you're placing bite-sized pieces on your fork and chewing; *taste* the food as it's located on different parts of your tongue and when you chew; and *feel* your emotions when eating and when you're done. Rather than rushing or engaging in another activity while you're eating, savor each bite. Look deeply into the life course of the food.

Notice feelings of contentment and gratitude. Use the practice chart to record what you became aware of directly before, during, and after eating mindfully.

Walking Meditation

Have you noticed yourself hunched over your laptop because you're working too hard, walking with your head down because you're feeling sullen, or moving around in bed because you can't settle? When your body is in one place and your mind is miles away, you are disconnected from what you're doing and from *who's* doing it. This is a by-product of the mind-body disconnection and source of our loneliness. It reinforces the belief that you're broken and need to be fixed.

Walking meditation is an awareness practice that uses mental, emotional, and physical experience to strengthen connection to the present moment. As such, it provides a means of bringing this awareness into your daily life. It teaches you how to walk the Middle Path as it brings into balance the extremes, from lethargy and agitation to peace and tranquility. It encourages you to remember your original goodness—your wholeness, your completeness. As in all meditations, walking meditation shines light on the workings of the mind and is considered a meditation in movement practice:

> The purpose of walking meditation is to not try to get anywhere except into the present moment—to walk not for the purpose of arriving at a destination but for the purpose of being fully present in every step. Walking meditation teaches you how to experience life as a process, not a goal. (Marotta 2013, 54)

There are several ways to practice walking meditation. In one, with slow and deliberate motion, you walk back and forth for ten to twenty steps in each direction, bringing attention to sensations in your feet and legs and movement of your body while breathing consciously. In another, you pay simultaneous attention to the experience of walking and your sensory experience, noticing, for example, the fragrant scent of the rose, the vibrant hue of the leaf, the sound of the bird, the texture of the stone, or the breeze on your face. You may walk steadily and slowly in one direction or stop for a while to take it all in and then divert from your intended direction.

You can turn walking wherever you are into a meditation practice. By tuning into the simple and yet wondrous act of walking, you connect to the fullness of the present moment and sense of wholeness. "If you feel happy, peaceful, and joyful while you are walking, you are practicing correctly. Be aware of the contact between your feet and the Earth. Walk as if you are kissing the Earth with your feet" (Nhat Hanh 1992, 28).

When you notice the balance, coordination, energy, attention, and strength required in the simple act of walking, a deep appreciation of your body arises. When you take in the sounds, hues, textures, touch, and warmth of your environment, even a clump of dirt or sound of your shoes touching the ground is treasured. When you walk on the earth, every step can feel nourishing and every moment becomes alive (Nhat Hanh 1976, 11).

In walking meditation, you bring bare attention to the act of walking—to what is actually happening in you and to you in the present moment. You turn attention to the sensations of walking in the body and how you are relating to the act of walking—if you're relating with resistance (e.g., if you're clinging to or avoiding the experience) or acceptance (e.g., if you're one with the experience). When the mind wanders, attention is brought back to the sensations of walking.

Formal Practice: Walking Meditation

This walking meditation brings slow and deliberate motion to walking back and forth for ten to twenty steps. You will need to find an unobstructed area, either indoors or outdoors, where you can walk your desired number of steps. Attention is on the sensation of walking, with breathing held in awareness and your gaze at the ground directly in front. In walking meditation, the object of attention is the sensation of walking, and your intention is to not get anywhere except into the present moment (Marotta 2013, 55–57).

As you practice walking meditation, bring awareness to movement, body sensations, feeling tone, thoughts, and emotions.

Movement. Stand in Mountain pose at one end of your space. Be aware of the contact of your feet to the ground and the feeling of balance as you stand tall like a tree, your lower body rooting to the earth and your upper body reaching toward the sky. Notice the intricacies of the simple act of standing balanced and upright.

Shift your weight to one foot as the other foot slowly rises from the ground. Notice sensations of lifting—heaviness or lightness, pulling or pushing. Slowly move your raised foot forward, feeling into sensations in your body. Notice sensations of forward movement—smooth or jerky, fast or slow. Place the heel of your forward foot on the ground and then your toes. Notice sensations of placing—balance or imbalance, equal or unequal weight distribution, and angle of your body. Shift your weight to the other foot as you raise your foot. Notice the sense of impermanence—the arising and passing of all things—as one foot is placed and the other foot rises. Note how there's a sense of nothing to hold on to as you surrender to the process.

Continue to move your lifted foot forward and place the heel and then the toes of your forward foot on the ground. When you reach the end of your walking space, slowly and consciously turn and walk in the opposite direction.

Body sensations. Feel sensations in the varying points of contact on the bottom of your feet; between your toes; and on your ankles, legs, shins, calves, knees, and thighs. Notice how the hips and hip joints, pelvis, and spine sway to the side. Pay attention to the breath in the belly—to the center of your body universe. Notice your shoulders, the subtle swing of the arms, and the movement in your wrists and hands as you feel the light touch of air or clothing on your skin. Notice the position of your chin as it's held square to the ground and your head—jaw, lips, eyes, forehead, skull, and brain.

Feeling tone. Notice pleasant, unpleasant, and neutral feelings without trying to cling to them or be averse to them.

Thoughts. Notice if you're clinging to or avoiding the experience by judging whether you like or don't like what's happening; whether your mind is wandering into planning, fantasizing, or obsessing; or whether your mind is dull or sleepy. Notice if you're identifying with the experience *and what happens* to your balance and movement when your mind is attentive versus distracted. When your mind has wandered, make a mental note, "thinking," and escort the mind back to the object of attention—walking.

Emotions. Notice your emotional state—happy, sad, irritated, bored, angry, or frustrated. Pay attention to how your emotions are impacting your movement. If you're feeling impatient, frustrated, or serene, do you move more quickly or slowly, more jerky or smooth? Without trying to change how you're feeling, simply acknowledge your feelings and return to the sensation of walking.

End in Mountain pose. On your final turn, stand in Mountain pose, feeling the connection to the earth and the balance of the body. Use the practice log to record your experience. To follow to the guided walking meditation practice, go to www.janettimarotta.com/meditations.

Practice Log 4: Formal Practice—Walking Meditation
What did you learn/how did you benefit?   What were your challenges/what interfered?

DAY 1

DAY 2

DAY 3

DAY 4

DAY 5

DAY 6

DAY 7

Practice Log 4: Informal Practice—Mindful Eating
Note the influence of eating mindfully.

DAY 1
DAY 2
DAY 3
DAY 4
DAY 5
DAY 6
DAY 7

Five

WORKING WITH THOUGHTS SKILLFULLY

Everything happens for you, not to you.

—BYRON KATIE

In chapter 5, I describe the relationship between thoughts and stress and ways to work with thoughts skillfully to move toward states of well-being. Our thoughts, emotions, and physiology reside within us as intimate triplets. When we think we've done something dumb, we're embarrassed and blush. When we ponder the loss of a loved one, we're sad and cry. When we reflect on a fun experience, we're happy and laugh. This chain reaction between thoughts impacting emotions impacting physiology forges the landscape of our mental, emotional, and physical health.

Thoughts and emotions create a cascade of events that lead to such diverse outcomes as resignation versus resolution, giving up versus showing up, or perceiving obstacles versus recognizing challenges. In turn, physical health can be compromised and impact our ability to make wise decisions. Statements such as, "It's my fault for waiting too long. I don't deserve to have a child," create a vicious cycle of defeat, despair, and indecision when now, more than ever, you need to be kind to yourself and affirm your worth.

Below is a poem I wrote when experiencing infertility that captures the impact of this life crisis on self-worth:

Wonder

No wonder I've had performance anxiety,
I thought I had to perform.
No wonder I've been lonely,
I felt I didn't belong.
No wonder I've stayed busy always doing,
I believed I wasn't enough.
No wonder I've owned the story,
I couldn't find the script.
No wonder I needed good and bad,
I had to take sides.
No wonder there was no wonder.

Breaking Free by Turning Toward

Buddhist psychology starts from the perspective that it is primarily the beliefs we have, and how tightly we hold on to them, that account for our mental suffering. Rather than trying to get rid of thoughts, it's learning how to see thoughts skillfully (Kornfield 2008, 146–47). By witnessing thoughts from a detached perspective, you are able to disentangle from them and see them as "mental formations"—random events like clouds in the sky, forming, dispersing, and disappearing from sight.

In Buddhist psychology, thoughts are considered events, not facts. As such, there is nothing defining about thoughts—nothing to identify with. You are *not* your thoughts. Rather than identifying yourself as infertile and questioning *why* this is happening to you, infertility becomes the issue, and the question becomes *how* to work with it. Infertility is not the obstacle; fertility is the challenge.

It's not about changing the situation but how you're relating to the situation. When difficult situations, like infertility, are viewed as a challenge rather than an obstacle, these situations provide an opportunity to learn and grow rather than serve as a reflection of worth. Success and failure do not define who you are.

Our conditioned nature is to grasp or cling to what we want, to avoid or be averse to what we don't want, or to be deluded, blinded by ignorance, which tells us to put our head in the sand: "What I don't know doesn't hurt me." Clinging may cause one person to not be able to stop treatment, avoidance may cause another person to be unable to explore treatment options, and delusion may cause yet another to deny a problem and not seek treatment at all.

Strongly held personal stories—assumptions or expectations of what *should* be happening, as opposed to acknowledgment of what is *actually* happening—get in the way of making sound decisions and recognizing what is truly important. Mindfulness teaches you to welcome what's here, regardless of the situation or circumstance. This challenges assumptions and opens the field to exploration and discovery. Whenever you find yourself stuck in perseverating thoughts, unable to move forward or caught in ambivalence, mindfulness instructs you to ask two fundamental questions: "What am I resisting?" and "How can I open up?"

Buddha recognized three truths of reality. I will discuss the initial truth now and the remaining two in later chapters. The first is *dukkha*, meaning suffering or dissatisfaction. Our inherent tendency is to expect life to be free of suffering, and when things go wrong, we react: "This shouldn't be happening! If only I didn't have to deal with this! This isn't fair!" Our resistance to the way life is causes us to cling (hold on to or ruminate), avoid (push away from or deny), or be deluded (ignore). This teaching is succinctly illustrated by meditation teacher and author Shinzen Young (2004, 84): "Pain times Resistance equals Suffering."

The antidote to suffering, then, is acceptance, meaning being with what is and not wishing it were different. It doesn't imply you need to like or endorse what's happening. It suggests acknowledging what's happening and then working with it. The situation is not the problem; it's your relationship to it, your resistance that's the problem. The process is one of letting go, meaning letting be: accepting things as they are, without grasping onto them or alternatively pushing them away—allowing events to run their course.

It's important to clarify that acceptance means being with what is, because trying to accept can add yet another level of suffering, as once again we're trying to get somewhere other than where we're at. Similarly, it's important to understand letting go means letting be, because trying to let go can also feel like something to strive for. So by simply being with what is occurring and letting things be, healing occurs.

When you were a child, did you ever play with a woven straw finger cuff? You insert each pointer finger as far as possible into both ends of this four-inch long, half-inch-wide tube. When you try to pull your fingers out, the tube constricts, and you're stuck. The puzzle is finding a way to escape from the clutches of the cuff. Steven Hayes (2005, 37), founder of Acceptance and Commitment Therapy (ACT), uses this activity to demonstrate how pushing or pulling against what's happening doesn't work: "The more you struggle, the more constricted your movements will be. If you let go of the struggle, the more freedom you have to make new choices." In this simple yet profound little puzzle, we find meaning in the wisdom of paradox: the harder you try, the more stuck you become.

This lesson can also be demonstrated through the metaphor of learning how to ski downhill. Our tendency is to instinctively lean back to slow down; however, it's by leaning forward that you slow down and maintain your balance. Paradoxically, by turning toward, rather than away, you maintain your balance and stay on course.

Mindfulness instructs you to get closer to distressing thoughts and disturbing emotions in order to move through them. Acknowledging the impact of infertility on your life and personal experience helps you to legitimize your feelings and then work with them. It's not about resolving infertility;

it's about *integrating* it. There will always be a sense of loss, and that can be OK. Over time, the loss lessens, and you've changed in ways that would have not otherwise been possible. For one, experiencing sadness, loss, hopelessness, helplessness, and the array of emotions inherent to infertility develops the ability to be truly empathic to others' struggles, which in turn enables you to be compassionate toward others as well as yourself.

Like most women I have worked with, letting go of the genetic tie was traumatic for me. It took months before I could consider third-party parenting. Even today, I occasionally find myself silently reacting to comments or situations that spotlight the absence of a genetic connection. But it's only momentary, and gratitude invariably steps in and takes its place.

Through the practice of mindfulness, it's not that you won't feel sad, angry, or even despondent if an IVF cycle or pregnancy fails, but you develop the capacity to be with your experience and call upon the inner resources to soften, heal, and renew. Mindfulness invites you to move into any difficult experience or circumstance, not by bracing yourself more tightly but by loving yourself more deeply. When you *lean into* the slippery slope of infertility with mindfulness, you become a working force in your own health and well-being and an agent of change.

From Looking to Seeing

The analogy of being struck by two arrows is used in one of the teachings of the Buddha, called the Arrow Sutta, to demonstrate the impact of thoughts on suffering. Buddha teaches that when struck by an arrow, we experience physical pain. The arrow represents the physical pain or physical manifestations of pain, such as tears or tightness in the chest from the inescapable events that happen in life. This is referred to as unavoidable suffering. But if we add mental pain to the suffering through negative self-talk—by taking what has happened personally (e.g., condemning ourselves for being such an idiot) or fearing the worse—this is like being struck by a second arrow. We now have two pains when there could have been just one. This is referred to as optional suffering. This Buddhist sutra is often used to illustrate the teaching: pain is inevitable, but suffering is optional.

Exercise: Power of Thoughts

Bring to mind the following real or imagined situation. Someone close to you just became pregnant after only trying a short amount of time. The news was delivered without any acknowledgment that this could be difficult to hear, given you've been trying for such a long time and there have been so many losses along the way, such as failed treatment attempts, miscarriages, upsetting diagnoses, or poor prognoses.

Unwholesome self-talk. Repeat the following or any other unwholesome messages you may conjure up on your own, then notice how you feel by tuning in to the consequence of this experience:

- "I can't believe she was so insensitive."
- "She's such a jerk."
- "I never want to see her again."
- "She was just trying to hurt me."
- "This isn't fair."
- "I feel like life is passing me by."
- "I'll never get pregnant."

Wholesome self-talk. Repeat the following or any other wholesome messages you may invoke yourself, then notice how you feel by tuning in to the consequence of this experience:

- "I don't know why she didn't acknowledge my situation, but maybe she wasn't able for whatever reason."
- "She's been a friend of mine in the past and can be a friend again sometime later."
- "I can keep my distance for now and choose to say something or not."
- "I know she wasn't trying to hurt me."
- "I can get support from those who can empathize."
- "All things shall pass."
- "I can breathe through the upset."
- "I know I will have a child, somehow."

Were you able to sense the difference in the level of distress when telling yourself unwholesome thoughts that imposed resistance on the experience versus telling yourself wholesome thoughts that brought acceptance into the experience?

Reframing the Journey

When you see the world with an overlay of judgment, it's like looking through a pair of glasses with a dirty lens. We're so familiar with seeing through the smudges, we don't even notice they're there. After the glasses are cleaned, it's hard to believe how much crisper everything looks. But within a short amount of time, the splotches start building up, and we've grown accustomed to them once again.

Viewing through a judgmental lens means perceiving concepts or interpretations that are not actually true or valid. So often, these interpretations lead to unwholesome thoughts—intrusive, distorted thoughts that create distressing emotions and gloomy moods. But when you view the world through nonjudgmental awareness in the present moment, your bare attention is on what is actually occurring in *real time*. You're able to notice unwholesome thoughts from past regrets or future worries and invite wholesome thoughts from the present to arise.

Western psychology defines *cognitive distortions* as negative, intrusive, invalid thoughts that create disturbing feelings and *cognitive reframes* as thoughts that accurately portray the situation and lead to emotions that create positive feelings. The specific therapeutic model that focuses on the role of thoughts to change the way we think, feel, and behave is known as cognitive behavior therapy (Burns 1990). The aim is to actively and directly change the way you think. Dr. Burns lists ten cognitive distortions, which include the following (1980, 42–43):

- All-or-nothing thinking; overgeneralizing (interpreting an event as part of an endless pattern of defeat).
- Obsessing on the negatives; dismissing the positives; expanding things out of proportion or shrinking their importance.
- Reasoning based on feelings; criticizing yourself or others.

- Labeling yourself a flawed person in some way; berating yourself for what you *should* have done.

Mindfulness uses the cornerstone quality of acceptance to recognize things as they are and reduce your resistance to them. Acceptance stands strong among the seven "pillars of mindfulness" identified by Jon Kabat-Zinn (1990, 31–41).

> Acceptance is a practice of getting curious—discovering what causes you to feel uncomfortable. It's the essential paradox of turning things around—moving toward that which you resist. In order to do this, you bring to bear the qualities of nonjudging, nonstriving, beginner's mind, letting be, and patience. These interrelated qualities…build upon one another and culminate in a greater capacity for trust as self-reliance: being able to rely on your mind and body through deep connection. (Marotta 2013, 6)

Trying to fix who you are or what you're thinking or feeling is not the intention of mindfulness, because this would be practicing nonacceptance. The way change occurs is a fundamental difference between Western and Buddhist psychology. The paradoxical approach of mindfulness uses acceptance as an essential agent of change and believes change innately arises through insight and awareness. Here we meet another mindfulness paradox: when not trying to change, change naturally occurs. Because mindfulness takes the judgment out of experience, cognitive reframes are an inherent consequence.

To reiterate, mindfulness places attention not on the stressor (because you are not spending energy on deciding whether the situation is bad or good or whether you want it to occur or not) but rather on how you're relating to it. For example, how are you emotionally relating to the thought (e.g., fueling the thought with fear or anxiety)? What is the energy (relationship) behind the thought (e.g., clinging to the thought by obsessing or ruminating)? How are you physically manifesting the thought (e.g., holding tightness in your chest or feeling your heart pounding)?

Mindfulness encourages testing the validity of thoughts by asking yourself, "Is this thought really true?" Exploring where thoughts come from by tracing them back to your childhood, past events, or circumstances deepens understanding and promotes insight.

Exercise: Inviting Wholesome Thoughts to Arise

The following exercise integrates models from Western and Buddhist psychology to work with thoughts skillfully.

Step 1: *Unwholesome thought.* Identify a chronic, unwholesome, pervasive thought that creates feelings of distress relating to your challenge with fertility. Write this thought on a piece of paper.

Step 2: *Witness.* Observe what *emotion* is fueling the thought. Observe the *energy* behind the thought. Observe how the *body* is manifesting the thought and feeling.

Step 3: *Inquire.* Where does this thought come from? Does it have roots in your childhood, your family of origin, a traumatic event, or circumstance? Is this thought true? How do you know it's true?

Step 4: *Wholesome thought.* Listen for a kinder, gentler, truer thought to emerge that affirms what you are doing or how you are attempting to move forward.

Step 5: *Witness.* Observe what *emotion* is fueling the thought. Observe the *energy* behind the thought. Observe how the *body* is manifesting the thought and feeling.

Exercise: Reframe Reminders

Write your wholesome thought on an index card as a reminder to take this thought with you into everyday life. Place your card where it's easily seen or within reach, such as on the refrigerator door, bathroom mirror, edge of the computer monitor, back of a cell phone, or inside your purse. If you find yourself lapsing into your unwholesome thought, refer to your card to support the truth of your reframe. Whenever you discover another unwholesome thought, invite wholesome thoughts to arise and add what you've uncovered to your posting of index cards.

Reframe Examples

Below are examples from women and men I have worked with who have used this East-West model to reframe unwholesome thoughts into wholesome thoughts:

- *Unwholesome thought*: "I'm infertile because I'm stressing myself out. I think I'm responsible for my own infertility. I blame myself." *Wholesome thought*: "I'm taking action to manage my stress. I know rationally that infertility can be inexplicable (no fault.) I'm taking good care of myself. I believe that I am meant to be a parent. I just don't know when or how it will happen."
- *Unwholesome thought*: "Why is this happening to us?" *Wholesome thought*: "This may be about coming to terms with not knowing everything. But I do know that this process is bringing my wife and me closer."
- *Unwholesome thought*: "I feel worthless because I can't get pregnant." *Wholesome thought*: "I've tried alternative treatments. I'm looking at the bigger picture of my life. I'm taking care of myself and managing stress. Everything is happening for a reason, although I may not know why. Perhaps this is a challenge or a learning opportunity, which is opening me up—open to adoption and other alternatives."
- *Unwholesome thought*: (a woman with secondary infertility) "I am failing my husband and daughter." *Wholesome thought*: "I bring more to our life than childbearing. I am more than an infertility patient."
- *Unwholesome thought*: "I'm having trouble conceiving because I've waited too long. Am I just too old to achieve pregnancy?" *Wholesome thought*: "I'm more mature, and when I do become a parent, I'll be a more capable parent. Age is a distortion! I'm exploring and evaluating various options."
- *Unwholesome thought*: "I feel like a failure. Something is wrong with me. I don't deserve to be a mom, and I'm being punished." *Wholesome*

thought: "I am more than this experience. This is not the only thing I am. I have a lot to be proud of—I'm independent and self-reliant. I have made my own life and built a career."

- *Unwholesome thought*: "Before every cycle, I am worried I'm setting myself up for disappointment." *Wholesome thought*: "Every step I take in the process of fertility treatments brings me one step closer to my dream of motherhood. The process is a journey."

- *Unwholesome thought*: "I am afraid to be hopeful. I don't know what or where the answers are." *Wholesome thought*: "I am courageous, growing stronger, getting healthier, and taking care of myself. All of this grows hope and certainty. I know there is a child for me."

- *Unwholesome thought*: "It's not my fault we can't have a baby; it's his." *Wholesome thought*: "We're in this together and will figure this out together. Through this challenge, we're learning how to truly support each other."

- *Unwholesome thought*: "Things are never going to get any better." *Wholesome thought*: "I look at my fear, and I let it go, and what remains is love and hope."

Exercise: Visualization to Work with Thoughts

This visualization practice invites you to identify a thought that disempowers (unwholesome thought) and to uncover a thought deep inside that affirms your true worth (wholesome thought). As you settle into a comfortable position, gently close your eyes. Allow the breath to settle down to its own rhythm as you begin to ride upon the in-breath and out-breath.

Imagine walking in a lush emerald meadow with a carpet of soft grass, adorned in wildflowers of indigo and sapphire blues and surrounded by shimmering emerald trees. As you're exploring, you discover a magic pond. You are called to bring to your mind's eye a judgmental, distorted belief that leads to feelings of unworthiness. As you conjure up this distorted belief, it takes the form of a solid, heavy rock. You are compelled to throw the big rock into the pond, and it quickly sinks into the pool's bottomless depth.

A luminous ball gently begins to rise to the surface. Contained within is a true belief that recognizes your essential nature—your Buddha nature—your whole and complete self, just as you are. This ball is filled with your virtuous qualities and recognizes the actions you're taking to move forward on your journey. This is your core self, your truth, your perfection within your imperfection. Invite the glow of golden healing light from the luminosity of this truth to shine around and through you. Breathe into and out from the heart, absorbing its truth ever more deeply.

When ready to leave this magic pond and the beauty that surrounds, bow to its compassionate wisdom and carry the truth of your wholeness into the world.

Choiceless Awareness

Following meditation on the breath and meditation on the body comes meditation on thoughts—a practice with a framework to work with thoughts skillfully. Because this practice teaches how to inquire into thoughts without identifying with them, it's helpful to first learn to witness thoughts from a detached perspective, which weakens their hold.

Choiceless awareness opens the field of experience to include breath, body sensations, sound, and thoughts as *mental formations*, random events to simply witness. Attention moves to whatever sense is most predominant and then shifts when another sense draws your attention. When a thought becomes most prevalent, the thought itself becomes the object of attention. Rather than trying to investigate, judge, cling to, or distract yourself from the thought, you simply witness the thought as a cloud in the sky, coming and going, leaving no trace. You continue to effortlessly shift to whatever sensation is most predominant in that moment—into choiceless awareness.

Rather than trying to decide what sense to attend to, you invite the sense to choose you. No sense or sensation is seen as a distraction or something to change but rather an opening to intimate exploration and knowing. When your mind wanders, attention is brought back to whatever sensation enters the field of awareness. If at any time you feel too uncomfortable with any sensation, you return to the breath.

In his MBSR program, Kabat-Zinn (1990, 71) teaches a practice called meditation on the senses, which ends in choiceless awareness. You are first instructed to bring attention to the breath and then systematically to touch and body sensation, sound, thoughts, and lastly to choiceless awareness. By systematically choosing the object of attention, it can be easier to float in choiceless awareness, where the object chooses you.

Choiceless awareness exposes the reality of impermanence—how things change in their own time. When observing each sense in meditation with an open, neutral stance, you are able to more clearly witness life's transient nature. You learn to relinquish control and meet yourself and life occurrences in their natural unfolding. As in all meditations, this practice generalizes to the practice of life itself and in particular fosters flexibility, resilience, and courage.

Formal Practice: Choiceless Awareness

To begin the practice of choiceless awareness, anchor your attention on the breath or ground yourself in the body. When ready, open your field of awareness to include the breath, body sensation, sound, and thoughts, seamlessly shifting attention to whatever sense or sensation calls you. When your mind wanders, bring your awareness back to whatever sensation beckons your attention. Return to the breath if any sensation becomes too uncomfortable.

Breath. If the breath is most noticeable, ride upon the current of the breath, noticing the unique qualities of each breath.

Body Sensation. If body sensation is most dominant, feel ever more deeply what is here to be felt, noticing skin sensations, temperature variations, or density of the felt sensations and how sensations change and run their course.

Sound. If sound is most prevalent, listen ever more acutely to what is here to be heard, noticing how sound has a beginning, middle, and end and how sound is loud and soft, distant and near, high pitched and low pitched, with spaces in between.

Thoughts. If thoughts are most pronounced, witness thoughts as clouds in the sky coming and going, leaving no trace, noticing how thoughts weave stories that take on a life of their own and how, as you step back to witness thoughts as mental formations, they no longer transmute into your personal narrative. You are not the thought, and the thought is not you.

Record your experience of choiceless awareness in the practice log. What did the practice teach? How did you grow? What were your challenges? How did resistance show up? To listen to this guided meditation practice, go to www.janettimarotta.com/meditations.

Meditation on Thoughts

Now that you've practiced witnessing thoughts as mental formations coming and going, in this next meditation, when a dominant, intrusive, unwholesome thought emerges that refuses to leave, the thought itself becomes the object of attention for innermost exploration. Meditation on thoughts teaches how to see thoughts skillfully by naming the thought and thought pattern and investigating the emotion fueling the thought, the energy (relationship) behind the thought, and the physical manifestation of the thought.

As you learn to witness the thought stream from a detached, neutral perspective, you notice how these stories fall into familiar, repetitious thought patterns or tapes. Mental noting is used to neutralize the thought. This is represented in the well-known expression "Name it to tame it." First, you *name the thought.* If you find yourself lost in self-judgment, you state, "This is judging." Second, you *name the tape.* If you hear yourself saying, "I'll never have a child," you might label the tape "The Little Engine That Couldn't." Using a friendly label helps to befriend the thought and not see it as an enemy to eradicate. This perspective is captured in the phrase "What you resist persists."

Psychologist, insight-meditation teacher, and author Tara Brach popularized a way of investigating thoughts in meditation through the acronym RAIN: recognize, accept, investigate, nonidentify (2012, 61–75), which is outlined in the following meditation.

Formal Practice: Meditation on Thoughts

In meditation on thoughts, when a dominant, intrusive, unwholesome thought emerges, the thought itself is the object of attention. It is then investigated by using the RAIN practice. When your mind wanders, return to the object of attention—thoughts. Know that if you encounter too much distress during any time of this process, you may return to the breath to anchor and stabilize.

R = recognize the thought as it arises.

Name the thought as you recognize it through mental noting (e.g., "regretting"), saying to yourself, "This is regretting." Other possibilities may be judging, planning, resenting, or mistrusting. Name the tape when you notice a conditioned negative and pervasive thought pattern. Use a phrase that allows you to step back from it with humor or compassion (e.g., "Lost Horizon").

A = accept or allow the thought to be present, whatever it is.

Accept the thought by letting it move through you without clinging or avoiding.

I = investigate the thought through emotions, energy, and body sensations.

Observe the emotion that is fueling the thought, as this is the emotion that may make the thought repetitive and reinforce a never-ending pattern of defeat. For example, anxiety and fear stimulates rehearsing the future. Guilt and shame stimulates rehashing the past. Notice the effect of this emotion on mood.

Observe the energy (relationship) behind the thought; in other words, how are you relating to the thought—do you run, attach to, minimize, or deny?

Observe the body as it's manifesting the thought. The body speaks the truth and is more trustworthy than thoughts, which tend to weave stories that aren't even true. Where in your body do you feel the tension? What does it feel like?

N = *nonidentify* with the thought.

Nonidentify with the thought, allowing yourself to let go of judgment without clinging to or avoiding the thought. Rather than identifying with the thought as *mine*, observe it as a nonpersonal event—experience arising out of conditions and then passing away. Relax, breathe, and rest your awareness in compassion. End with the acknowledgment of your courage to embrace and work with what is present.

Along with the formal practice of choiceless awareness, record your meditation on thoughts in the practice log. Remember, charting your meditations is an especially helpful means of establishing and maintaining your practice. Establishing the practice by listening to each chapter's guided meditation (www.janettimarotta.com/meditations) can really help.

Informal Practice: Cognitive Awareness

Throughout the day, notice the impact of unwholesome versus wholesome thoughts on your emotional and physical well-being.

What unwholesome thought is connected to your emotion and the mood that develops? What is the energy behind the thought? How does the body manifest this thought-and-feeling connection? For example, you might notice how the thought "I'm being punished" is linked to the emotion of despair and how this is associated with a depressed mood; you're clinging to it with guilt, and your body feels tense.

What wholesome thought is connected to your emotion and the mood that develops? What is the energy behind the thought? How does the body manifest this thought-and-feeling connection? For example, you might notice how the thought "I know I will have a child if I open to possibility" is linked to the emotion of calm and how this is associated with a peaceful mood; your energy is open and accepting, and your body feels relaxed. Record your cognitive awareness in the practice log.

Practice Log 5: Formal Practice—Choiceless Awareness & Meditation on Thoughts
What did you learn/how did you benefit?   What were your challenges/what interfered?
DAY 1
DAY 2
DAY 3
DAY 4
DAY 5
DAY 6
DAY 7

Practice Log 5: Informal Practice—Cognitive Awareness

Note the influence of unwholesome versus wholesome thoughts on emotional and physical well-being.

DAY 1

DAY 2

DAY 3

DAY 4

DAY 5

DAY 6

DAY 7

Six

MAKING SPACE FOR EMOTIONS

*The "full catastrophe" captures something positive
about the human spirit's ability to come to grips
with what is most difficult in life and to find within
it room to grow in strength and wisdom.*

—JON KABAT-ZINN

We proceed from learning how to work with thoughts skillfully to learning how to work with emotions. Like thoughts, mindfulness does not identify an emotion as positive or negative but as having the potential to become destructive if resisted (in other words, if judged, obsessed over, avoided, or controlled). Mindfulness teaches to turn toward distressing emotions with the quality of openness: a wide, receptive, accepting state that can contain all things without limitation. Openness allows emotions to move through you without clinging to them or trying to avoid them. This is possible when you create space for emotions to be.

The analogy of salt in water is used in one of the teachings of the Buddha, called the Lonaphala Sutta, to explain how the practice of mindfulness helps you receive and hold difficult experiences. If a tablespoon of salt is added to a cup of water, the taste of salt is overpowering. But if a tablespoon of salt is added to a pond, the taste of salt is vastly diluted. Similar to salt in a pond, painful emotions disperse in a spacious, open heart. Life will be easier if you are open.

Most struggle with the recommendation of a third-party parenting option, fearing they won't bond with the child—that the child isn't really "theirs." But when moving through a fertility challenge with openheartedness, sadness and loss make room for kindness and gratitude, and you change in unexpected ways.

Many years ago, I heard the story of a father with an adopted son. When the son turned three years old, the mother learned quite by surprise that she was pregnant. When the father heard they were going to have another child, he said, "I only hope I love this child as much as I love the son we have!" With the quality of openness, "The heart has room for everything" (Levine 1979, 70).

Welcoming the Unwelcome

In Buddhist psychology, emotions are a response to all experience and arise as physical sensations in the body and thoughts in the mind. Like comrades on a joint mission, our thoughts construct stories, and our emotions confirm these stories are true. Within seconds, we fall down a rabbit hole and can't see the light of day. But emotions, like thoughts, are nonpersonal events arising out of conditions and then passing away. Emotions come and go; there is nothing to hold on to. And like thoughts, emotions are neither positive nor negative in themselves. They are referred to as pleasant, unpleasant, and neutral "feeling tones" that are just how our body and mind react to particular sensations.

Buddhist psychology identifies three underlying tendencies of mind that prevent us from seeing clearly and acting skillfully: greed (clinging), hatred (avoiding), and delusion (denying). Our inherent tendency is to want to feel good, to not feel bad, and to not see what's truly happening. Mindfulness teaches you to welcome distressing emotions and, like thoughts, observe how you relate to them, such as obsessing over them or minimizing or avoiding them. When letting in the uninvited guests, they will stay awhile and then pass through, like boats sailing on the river of tears and floating away. Rather than clinging to what you want or avoiding what you don't want and looking for short-term fixes, mindfulness points you in the direction of painful emotions so you can work with them and find long-term integration.

In one of the many allegories of Buddha, the demon Mara appears in different forms to derail Buddha off the path of enlightenment. In one story, Mara attempts to seduce Buddha away from spiritual life by sending his three striking daughters. But Buddha recognizes these women as representing thirst, desire, and delight and is not led astray. In another story, Mara tries to kill Buddha with an army who attacks with a fusillade of arrows. Buddha meets the test by transforming the shooting arrows into a shower of flowers. Rather than seeing Mara as an enemy, Buddha recognizes him as a teacher who tests his commitment and brings him insight into the nature of life, including potential traps. When Mara brings you a test, ask yourself these questions: "When Mara is my enemy, how do I shut down? When Mara is my teacher, how can I open up?"

Buddhist psychology identifies five powerful hindrances that influence emotions and thoughts. These hindrances take away our ability to see the big picture by seducing us into personal dramas and leading us to unwholesome action. It is important to understand the form each hindrance can take and how each hindrance can be neutralized:

- *Sensual desire*—compulsive wanting (clinging, e.g., obsessing over what you want) and neutralized by committing to your intention.
- *Ill will*—not wanting something (aversion, e.g., pushing others away with critical, judgmental behavior) and neutralized by exploring your beliefs and speaking from your heart.

- *Sloth and torpor*—laziness and boredom (e.g., losing interest because you're not actively engaged) and neutralized by quieting your mind to investigate what you're resisting.
- *Restlessness and worry*—wanting things to be different (clinging to pleasure and avoiding pain, e.g., distracting yourself from your intention) and neutralized by moving into your feelings of discomfort to feel more connected.
- *Doubt*—losing faith or becoming disheartened (e.g., questioning commitment to your intention) and neutralized by understanding your feelings and using your strengths to carry you through.

As an observer of emotions, you learn to notice your unwholesome emotional reactions and the consequences of these emotions to your behavior so you can mindfully choose to respond with wholesome actions. Mindfulness teaches how to unhinge from conditioned, pervasive, and unwholesome emotionally reactive patterns and be guided by wisdom and insight. In this process, emotional maturity grows.

Meditation on Emotions

In the previous meditations, awareness is brought to different objects of attention, such as breath, body sensations, and thoughts. But when an emotion becomes so pronounced that it becomes difficult to stay with the object of attention, the emotion itself becomes the object. Examining the emotion that arises in meditation can help you see what is wholesome and unwholesome and work with it.

Mindfulness makes room for whatever is here, without judgment, evaluation, clinging, or aversion. When you explore an emotion, you investigate three expressions of the emotion. What *thoughts* are connected to your emotion (e.g., is there a judgmental statement you tell yourself)? What *energy* (relationship) is behind the emotion (e.g., do you run from, attach to, minimize, or deny)? How does the *body* manifest the emotion (e.g., is there physical tightness or constriction)? Can you then simply witness the emotion and let it be?

If investigating the emotion becomes overly stressful, come back to the breath to calm and center. You can then choose to return to the emotion or know you've gone far enough and let it be. Similar to meditation on thoughts, when practicing meditation on emotions, it's helpful to use the acronym RAIN: recognize, accept, investigate, nonidentify.

Formal Meditation: Meditation on Emotions

In meditation on emotions, when an intrusive emotion emerges that won't seem to let go, the emotion itself becomes the object of attention and is then investigated by using the RAIN practice. When your mind wanders, return to the object of attention—emotions. Know if you encounter too much distress during any time of this process, return to the breath to anchor and stabilize.

Recognize the emotion as it arises using mental noting (e.g., "sadness"), saying to yourself, "This is sadness." Naming helps you to avoid identifying with and entangling in the emotion.

Allow the emotion by letting it move though you—without clinging to the emotion or avoiding it.

Investigate how your emotion is tied to your thoughts (e.g., is judgment in the thought—a critical statement that sets a tone or mood?), what the energy is behind the emotion (e.g., do you cling, avoid, or deny the emotion and what feelings are attached, e.g., guilt, remorse, or shame?), and how the body is manifesting the emotion (e.g., is there physical tightness or constriction, cold or flush of heat, trembling or numbness and where are these sensations stored, e.g., in your solar plexus, head, or shoulders?). What happens to the shape, tone, and intensity of the emotion as you observe it in your thoughts, moods, and body?

Nonidentify with the emotion, moving into it as an explorer. Ask yourself, for example, "What is sadness?" Without clinging to or avoiding the emotion or identifying with the emotion as *mine*, observe it as a nonpersonal event—experience arising out of conditions and then passing away. Use the breath to move into the emotion, creating space for the emotion to dissipate or simply be. Hold the emotion in compassion. End with the acknowledgment of your courage to embrace and work with what is present.

Record your experience in the practice log, noticing the space you're creating for emotions to settle and soften. Use the guided meditation on emotions to help you establish this practice located on my website: www.janettimarotta.com/meditations.

Informal Practice: Emotional Awareness

Emotions and thoughts are linked not only to physiology but also to our actions. Throughout the day, notice the impact of this interplay among emotions, thoughts, physiology, and actions. What thought is connected to your emotion and the mood that develops? What is the energy behind the emotion? How does the body manifest this emotion? How does this mind-body interchange control your actions? What actions allow more space? For example, you might notice how the emotion of sadness is linked to the thought, "I'm a failure," and how this thought is associated with a depressed mood; you're clinging to it with regret, your body feels dull and tired, and you react by shutting down and watching television. Then you might notice actions that allow more space include taking a walk or sitting down to meditate. Record your emotional awareness in the practice log.

The Grieving Process

If there is one word to describe infertility, it's "loss." There may be multiple miscarriages, failed IVFs, or unexpected medical test results. Next month's period can feel like yet another loss. There is loss in relationships, emotional well-being, time, and money. There is loss of a life well lived and "loss of a dream."

Our conditioned model of control is driven by the belief that life should be free of suffering and permanently remain comfortable and certain. As loss grows over time, so does a sense of insecurity, in part because loss is internalized as a lost sense of self. Yet it's not so much the loss that's feared but the life there is to live.

The problem with this model of control is exemplified in Buddha's three truths of reality. We discussed Buddha's first truth, *dukkha*, meaning dissatisfaction. It's our resistance to the inherent dissatisfactory nature of life that causes suffering. Buddha labeled the second characteristic of existence *anicca*, or impermanence. Our need to have all our "ducks in a row" causes us to resist the fact that all things change. Ultimately, we have no control, but we fight against it. We then tend to personalize experience and try to prove that we're permanently OK, resisting the third truth of reality, *anatta*, or no self (discussed in the next chapter).

To stop fighting against the lack of control over your situation with fertility, you need now more than ever to cultivate patience—the understanding that some situations unfold in their own time, outside your control. You come to understand the wisdom in patience through the saying, "There is nothing that's permanent except impermanence—nothing remains without change" (Kung 2006, 5).

Many fear emotions will become so overwhelming that they will drown in their tears. Attempts to become pregnant take on a life of their own, and a race against time is set in motion. But ironically, it's a race from the very tears needed to sustain the journey. Renowned Buddhist nun and author Pema Chodron (2000, 32) writes, "The most fundamental aggression to ourselves, the most fundamental harm we can do to ourselves, is to remain ignorant by not having the courage and the respect to look at ourselves honestly and gently."

In the classic book *On Death and Dying* (1969), Kubler-Ross identifies five stages of the grieving process: denial and isolation, anger, bargaining, depression, and acceptance. She asserts that only when you pass through the first four stages can you find acceptance. While there are differences in dynamics, development, and intensity, the inherent loss embedded in the infertility experience has been described as similar to these stages (Cooper-Hilbert 1998, 39–46; Deveraux and Hammerman 1998, 110–15).

These stages are currently viewed by experts in the field of loss and grief as states that rise and fall in no predictable linear form: "Grief and anger aren't extinguished like flames doused with water. They can flicker away one moment and burn hot the next" (Sandberg and Grant 2017, 55). See if you can relate to these states of grief:

- *Denial and isolation.* It's not unusual to deny that a fertility problem exists and to become paralyzed to make an appointment with a fertility clinic or wait beyond a reasonable amount of time. Avoidance, minimization, procrastination, and numbness are faces of denial. Feeling isolated and alone is a predominant feeling.
- *Anger.* Infertility often leads to feelings of anger toward the situation, yourself, or your partner. Anger can manifest in feelings of resentment toward the situation or a sense of unfairness in being singled out: "It's not fair!" Jealousy or envy at others' pregnancies follow, along with a sense of being disconnected or misunderstood by others who can't understand, empathize, or support.
- *Bargaining.* Bargaining is recognized as attempts to force a desired outcome when it's not necessarily in your best interest. It may appear in the form of obsessing over fertility treatment, pursuing multiple options at the same time, believing pregnancy is the only solution, extending treatment beyond repeated recommendations, or being stuck in confusion.
- *Depression.* When hope or belief in someday having a child is lost, becoming consumed by depression and despair ensues. Emptiness, sadness, feelings of inferiority, exhaustion, or stress-related symptoms may follow.
- *Acceptance.* Emotions present the necessary fodder that allows you to let go and find acceptance—the ability to be with the situation as it

is, without forcing it to be otherwise. Acceptance can be seen when you're able to

- ° talk about infertility without guilt, shame, or hopelessness,
- ° relinquish control as your major coping mechanism,
- ° understand the importance of parenting over genetics,
- ° find agreement and support with your partner,
- ° be willing to be educated about family-building options,
- ° believe you will have a child if you're open to possibility,
- ° become an active participant in your own healing journey.

Mindfulness uses nonjudgmental awareness to meet any and all situations, including grief, and begins by acknowledging what you are feeling. Acknowledgment alone produces change, as opening to what is occurring without wishing it away enables space for feelings to run their course or simply be. This nonjudgmental approach opens the door for seeking help and sharing emotions with understanding confidants. This lessens isolation, depression, hopelessness, and feelings of being burdened. Expressing loss allows feelings to be present and ultimately soften, making space for new coping resources to emerge.

While loss is rooted in every pregnancy attempt, it also provides information on what step to take next. A failed IVF can determine whether it's worth trying again or if it's time to move to egg donation. While the range of emotions connected to infertility can feel harsh and unrelenting, one emotion leads to another and can open you up in unexpected ways. Sorrow can give rise to compassion, and compassion can awaken gratitude. The gratitude you find when you finally do have a child will make you the parent you might not have become otherwise.

Infertility represents a crisis because of its overwhelming impact on all areas of life. Crisis has the potential to draw out your worst or elicit your best, as crisis represents both danger and opportunity. Chinese philosopher Confucius pronounced, "Our greatest glory is not in never falling, but in rising every time we fall." When actively engaged in the grieving process, the inner resources you discover become the gift of a lifetime. You begin to understand that every loss brings you a step closer to your child.

WORKING WITH GRIEF

Awareness leads to insight, from which change innately arises because you are able to recognize what leads to suffering (how you get stuck) and what leads to non-suffering (how you break free). You begin to notice the cause-effect relationship between the interplay of thoughts, emotions, and physical feelings on your actions. Mindfulness takes you out of reactivity mode so you can consciously choose how to respond. Because it's an active process, it's integrally filled with possibility and change. To move through grief, it too needs to be an active process. Below are examples of intentional actions recognized to be helpful for "griefwork." As you explore these possibilities, record your experience in your journal.

Notice thoughts, and work with them skillfully. When you experience a difficult emotion, investigate the thought behind the emotion. Ask yourself, "Am I blaming myself or others, failing to acknowledge my efforts and qualities, or predicting the worst to happen?" Are you saying statements like, "I don't deserve to get pregnant and never will"? Conversely, are you accepting or allowing the thought; investigating the emotions, energy, and physical sensations tied to this thought; and nonidentifying with the thought as a statement of personal worth? Whatever wholesome thought arises, write it on an index card to be reminded of your true self, your original goodness.

Make room for emotions and notice patterns. Notice if you have a pattern of behavior, such as minimizing, isolating, keeping busy, waiting for time to pass, saying you're OK when you're not, or comparing yourself to others. Identify unwholesome patterns by asking yourself three primary questions:

1. "What am I feeling?" (e.g., sadness). "What thoughts, mood, and attitudes are associated?" (e.g., "I'll never get pregnant" along with a depressed mood or hopeless attitude). "How is my body holding the emotion?" (e.g., back and shoulder pain).
2. "How is this emotional cascade controlling my actions?" (e.g., withdrawing).
3. "What actions allow healing?" (e.g., calling a friend).

Identify triggers. Identify statements from others that don't feel helpful. In the case of secondary infertility, this might include, "At least you already have a child. Be grateful for what you have." For primary infertility, it could be, "It wasn't meant to be. Time will heal. Just relax—go on vacation. Just adopt—then you'll have a child."

Consider letting others know what they can say that would be helpful to hear. You might suggest it seems like they're trying to be helpful, but what you really need from them is to *just listen*.

Employ mindful communication. Most couples don't know how to support each other when both are hurting and coping styles conflict. Because sharing grief with your partner is vital to the grief process, use *wise listening* and *wise speech* (described in chapter 8) to form the basis of your communication.

Invite support. Obtain support from others who can relate to or understand your grief. Joining a fertility group offers emotional support and a sense of not being alone in your grief. Pursuing individual or couples counseling, ideally from a therapist who specializes in fertility, can help guide you through the healing process. Seek information and support via websites, books, and fertility organizations. The website ihr.com lists all national nonprofit infertility organizations. For example, RESOLVE provides information and support for infertility, and SANDS is a support group for those who have experienced miscarriage, stillbirth, or neonatal death. Refer to the resources in the back of the book for links to other helpful organizations. Support yourself by taking breaks from treatment for healing and renewal.

Rituals have been used throughout the centuries in all parts of the world to acknowledge loss and offer closure. Plan a ritual alone or with your partner that symbolically represents your loss. This may take the form of planting a tree or floating a message in a bottle out to sea.

Practice Log 6: Formal Practice—Meditation on Emotions

What did you learn/how did you benefit?   What were your challenges/what interfered?

DAY 1
DAY 2
DAY 3
DAY 4
DAY 5
DAY 6
DAY 7

Practice Log 6: Informal Practice—Emotional Awareness

Note the influence of the interplay between emotions, thoughts, physiology, and actions.

DAY 1

DAY 2

DAY 3

DAY 4

DAY 5

DAY 6

DAY 7

Seven

MEETING CHALLENGING SITUATIONS

Be the change you want to see in the world!

—GANDHI

In chapter 7, I draw attention to identifying and uncovering ways to work with challenging interpersonal situations on the infertility path, as there is a complex array of circumstances that are frequently confusing, awkward, and painful. When receiving an invitation to yet another baby shower, do you support your friend or protect yourself? Do you tell your family and friends you're trying to become pregnant or keep it private? How do you manage doctor's appointments, surgeries, and procedures without disclosing to your employer that you're pursuing fertility treatment?

Comments often bring a barrage of reactions. You may feel minimized when you hear, "You just need to relax," imposed upon when asked, "Any news?" disregarded when never asked, "How are you doing?" or hurt when advised, "It's God's will."

Ironically, the people you typically received support from may now be the very ones who cause the most pain, and the places and activities you found most enjoyable may now be the ones you're least likely to visit or pursue. As exposure to these situations increases over time, the ability to cope often decreases, and a pattern of avoidance and retreat may then develop.

These are among the host of interpersonal challenges that keep the stress response on a constant low-grade red alert. How could it be otherwise when there's no way to predict exactly when or where these stressful events will rear their heads?

Being the Change Itself

For the most part, people are not able to understand the impact of infertility unless they have experienced it themselves. Comments tend to minimize the experience because infertility is not understood as the crisis it is. Though these comments are often interpreted as insensitive, they are almost always not intended to be so.

To meet these challenging situations, a particularly helpful quality to cultivate is beginner's mind or *don't know mind*: looking at things as if for the first time, without assumptions. When not making assumptions and interpretations, you are less likely to take things personally. Beginner's mind protects you from stepping on interpersonal land mines along the way. When a stressful comment or situation occurs, you say, "Don't know," and encounter it as the impersonal comment it actually is. Beginner's mind is fostered with an attitude of curiosity. By taking a curious, neutral stance, you are better able to concentrate not on the results but on the work itself. When not trying to change the situation, *you* become the change yourself.

The Comparing Mind

We tend to compare ourselves against others and have a need to "fit in"—to be like everyone else. In Buddhist psychology, this inherent tendency is referred to as the *comparing mind*. Because infertility is so personally threatening, this tendency manifests in spades. When the rest of the world seems to easily enter the very stage of life you so desire, it's impossible to not compare and, as a result, experience infertility as a personal failing.

Buddhist psychology emphasizes that clinging produces suffering. When obsessing on anything, we're holding on to concepts—ideas, perceptions, interpretations, fabrications, assumptions—which lead us to fall victim to the comparing mind. Concepts are the way we perceive things, and when caught by concepts, we become caught in our personal story. For example, if you are unable to become pregnant, you might believe it's because you're not deserving or that God is punishing you. If you hear that another friend is pregnant, you might label yourself a "bad person," because instead of being happy for your friend, you're feeling guilty for experiencing jealousy or envy.

Following what Buddha defines as the first truth of reality, *dukkha* (suffering or dissatisfaction), and the second truth of reality, *anicca* (impermanence), comes the third truth of reality, *anatta*, or *no self*. Our tendency is to secure a permanent sense of self that superimposes assumptions of who you are or who you *should* be onto what is actually happening. It's these concepts of self, or *ego*, that cause us to personalize experience through the lens of me, mine, and I. This automatically constructs a defensive position where you operate in me versus them mode. But in actuality, you are always changing. Nothing is fixed in time; nothing is solid. Rather, there is an ever-fluctuating flow of experience. There is *no self*—no fixed, permanent, solid self.

When you accept yourself, just as you are, the boundaries between *self* and *others* dissolve. In this space between, there is *no self*. When you let go of the ego, "egolessness" arises. We meet this paradox: "in the very process of knowing *self*, you lose *self*, and gain the world." As you learn to let go of the assumptions and interpretations that falsely define and confine your sense of self (ego), you become part of a much greater reality. You are part of the world and the world is part of you: "nothing is everything!"

When you notice that you have the tendency to superimpose your construct of self on top of what is happening, identify this as the ego being wounded by a series of expectations and assumptions based on external comparison.

Recognize your *wounded ego* and greet it at the front door! "Ah, here you are again, my suffering soul. I know you well!"

Meeting Trying Comments

As an awareness practice, mindfulness sheds light on how you get stuck and how you break free. You become aware of what behaviors and patterns lead to feelings that disaffirm worth and what actions honor your original goodness—your whole and complete self, just as you are. When difficult interactions occur and you notice a resulting feeling of distress and pattern of withdrawal or unhealthy behavior, notice what actions heal and soothe.

Employ beginner's mind. Along the infertility terrain, it's nearly universal to feel hurt by something that someone has said—or not said. At the ground floor of these encounters lies a foundation of judgment—judgment toward others and judgment toward yourself. Cultivating the quality of beginner's mind ("don't know" mind) becomes a wise ally. Good times to employ beginner's mind include, for example, when friends or family have not reached out to provide support or when others have said something that minimizes, interprets, or advises in unhelpful ways. Beginner's mind invites the possibility that comments have been expressed not from a place of *uncaring* but *unknowing*—being unaware of what to say, feeling afraid of saying the wrong thing, or not wanting to intrude on your privacy. When you employ "don't know" mind, you let go of assumptions and are thus better able to give others (and therefore yourself) the benefit of doubt. You free yourself from taking comments personally and heal the wounds that bind you.

Invite support. Reach for support from those who can understand and empathize. This might be from a sensitive friend, a family member who has experienced infertility, a counselor who specializes in fertility challenges, or a fertility support or mind-body group where you don't feel alone in what you're experiencing.

Remember the wise pause. When taking the *wise pause*, choice is possible. Take a few deep breaths, notice what you're thinking and how you're feeling, and bring back your attention to your body to calm and center. You've disengaged from reactivity mode and can now consciously choose how you wish to respond.

Choose your communication options.

- Communicate your feelings: When someone says, "You just need to relax," communicate how you're truly feeling (e.g., "It's not just about relaxing. I know you're trying to be helpful, but it hurts to hear that").
- Communicate the facts: Comments such as "why don't you just adopt?" are often based on false facts. Provide information by saying something like, "Do you know how hard it is to adopt? Couples compete with one another for babies to adopt. Adoption can cost thousands of dollars and take years."
- Communicate when ready: If you're not able to directly address an interaction, have an exit strategy, physically (e.g., leave the situation) and verbally (e.g., shift attention away from yourself). If you receive an e-mail or phone call, don't respond until you're ready, if at all. Tell yourself, "These are my feelings and they're legitimate." Saying no or intentionally sidestepping can be an act of self-compassion, as opposed to avoidance, if you're consciously choosing how to take care of yourself to your current best ability.

Choose your response in advance. It can be helpful to know what to say in advance of when you hear comments that feel hurtful or disaffirming. Below is a list of responses to commonly heard comments from women and men with whom I've worked.

"Any news?"

- "Trust me. When I'm pregnant, you'll know about it."
- "I know you're trying to be helpful, but…"

- "We're working on it."
- "I'll let you know when I'm ready."
- "We're having a baby when the time is right."

"You just need to relax!"

- "If only it was just about relaxing."
- "Relaxing doesn't cure infertility, like relaxing doesn't cure cancer."
- "Sometimes fertility issues need medical treatment, which is what we're doing."
- "Have you ever tried to relax in the middle of a crisis?"

"Why don't you just adopt?"

- "Are you offering yours?"
- "Do you know any that are available?"
- "Do you know how hard it is to adopt?"
- "We're pursuing one option at a time."

"It's God's will."

- "How do you know?"
- "We're not stopping here; some way we'll have a child—that's what God told us."
- "It's not that simple—God works in mysterious ways."

"I'm pregnant!"

- "I'm happy for you, but sometimes it might be hard for me to talk about it."
- "Congratulations."

- Tell yourself, "Their being pregnant has nothing to do with my chances of being pregnant."

"What's taking so long—when are you going to start a family?"

- "I have two dogs; they're my kids."
- "We already are a family."
- "We're trying, and we'll let you know when it happens."

"At least you can get pregnant."

- "I still don't have a baby."
- "You don't get credit for trying."
- "It really doesn't matter until there's a baby in my arms."
- "Having a miscarriage is a deep loss. It's not about just starting again."

"Oh, you'd be such a good mother!"

- "You're right! I will be a good mother."

"Why aren't you drinking?" (At a social event.)

- "I'm just not feeling like it tonight."
- "I'm the designated driver."

"At least you have one child." (Secondary infertility.)

- "There's nothing wrong with wanting more."
- "At least you have one leg!"
- "One's not enough to support us in old age!"
- "We feel siblings are really important."

"You're lucky you can go to the movies, get your nails done." (Someone with a child.)

- "Trade ya."
- "I'm lucky, and so are you."

Encountering Difficult Circumstances

As you learn to befriend yourself through the practice of mindfulness, you become your own best advocate. Below is a list of suggestions for commonly experienced difficult circumstances from those I've worked with clinically:

Impact on lifestyle

- Make taking care of yourself your number-one priority.
- Get together with others who produce feelings of positivity and participate fully in activities that bring you pleasure or that you may have always wanted to do.
- Eat a well-balanced diet, full of vegetables, fruit, and whole-grain foods (not processed or artificial ingredients), and limit caffeine and alcohol. This is a great diet to have now *and* the rest of your life.
- Maintain balance and moderation in everything you do.
- Keep a gratitude journal, bond with an animal, and practice generosity.

Life on hold

- Focus on the process rather than the goal of pregnancy—on the qualities you are cultivating.
- Practice gratitude. Focus on those things you do have, on the inside and outside.
- Reach out to others at times of need.
- Think of it this way: life is a fast-moving train, and you don't want to miss out on the ride!

Being surrounded by pregnant women

- Use the breath to calm and the body to ground and center.
- Have a handful of topics to discuss.
- Have an exit strategy.
- Seek support—contact your fertility group or someone close.

Whether to tell the family

- Every family situation and dynamic is unique, with different sets of rules and expectations. If your family is supportive, tell them. If your family is judgmental, don't tell them.
- Write a pros and cons list.

How to cope with holidays, celebrations, and missed milestones

- Do something else during the holidays, such as take a vacation.
- Cultivate compassion by helping others; for example, serve holiday dinner at a shelter.
- Create a ritual recognizing something special or meaningful.
- Say no to a baby shower and yes to taking care of yourself. Be true to yourself.
- Decide whether to go to events in advance.
- Have an exit strategy.

Work situations such as having to leave for appointments

- Change the work situation, if possible.
- Schedule medical appointments before work.
- Explain your situation to a manager or coworker, if appropriate.
- Be sure to receive clinic calls on your cell phone.
- Ask the nurse or doctor to hold and go outside for the call.
- Try to arrange to work from home for important calls, such as pregnancy outcome.

Dealing with others' judgment about third-party parenting

- Explain advanced reproductive technology.
- Try to reason.
- Choose to ignore.

Dealing with the complexity of decisions

- Discuss options with your partner and others.
- Brainstorm possibilities with your fertility group.
- Prep the discussion with information to draw from.

Not having an advocate

- Have someone in your corner who can help.
- Make a list of questions for every doctor's appointment.
- Educate yourself as best as you can. Become your own best advocate.

Journal: Challenging Situations

Identify two challenging situations that occurred with a colleague, friend, or family member, where you responded with unwholesome versus wholesome actions. In one situation, identify how you felt and how you shut down (responded with unwholesome actions). In the other situation, identify how you felt and how you opened up (responded with wholesome actions). Record these challenging situations in your journal.

Intentions of Well-Being

When twenty positive or neutral events and one negative event occurs during the day, we instinctively zero in on the negative one. What's happening here? Neuropsychologist and mindfulness teacher Rick Hanson (2009) describes the brain as "negativity biased." Our hardwired survival mechanism is conditioned to protect, defend, and be alert to what can go wrong. Hanson equates negative experiences sticking to the brain like Velcro and positive ones sliding off like Teflon. Given this hardwired mechanism, asserts Hanson, we need to intentionally "savor" the positive.

Fortunately, we have not only the relaxation response to counteract the stress response but also the "tend and befriend" response—our instinctive nature to protect our offspring and give and receive nurturance. It's the neurotransmitter oxytocin, "the hormone of love and bonding," that stimulates this response and calms emotional distress. This innate ability is evident in how we intuitively soothe ourselves when we rub a throbbing head or fan a sweaty face. Leading scientific expert on self-compassion Kristin Neff asserts our inherent biological nature demonstrates that "our brains are actually designed to care" (2011, 44).

To meet these challenging situations, cultivating self-compassion is a great benefactor. Self-compassion means caring for yourself in the same way you would care for someone you love. Self-compassion and compassion for others are cultivated in a number of Buddhist practices. They all draw upon sending intentions of wishing wellness to others. These "intentions of well wishing" help you cross from where you are in this present moment to where you *intend* or aspire to be.

Intentions are a powerful teaching in Buddhist psychology. When you take the *wise pause*, having clear intentions on how you wish to respond informs and guides your actions. By placing your attention on the present moment and your intention on how you're relating to the situation, you are reestablishing the cause-effect nature of life. You put your faith not on the outcome but on the process.

Insight-meditation teacher and author Gil Fronsdal describes how "mindfulness places us where choice is possible" and explains that the greater our intentions, the easier it is to choose what to do (2001, 60). He explains that "intentions are sometimes called seeds." Just like the garden we grow depends on the seeds we plant and water, the intentions we nurture condition our future happiness or unhappiness. If we water the seeds of our intentions with greed or hatred, pain and suffering will sprout and grow. If we water the seeds of our intentions with love or generosity, happiness and compassion will be nurtured and become a greater part of our life (2001, 61).

Exercise: Seeds of Intention

Turning the metaphor of seeds of intentions into an exercise with actual seeds demonstrates the cause-effect relationship between intentions and consequences. Take some seeds and plant them in a little pot of dirt. Place your pot where the sun can shine on it, nurture it with water, and watch its development with curiosity and fondness. Make an intention to care for the seeds as best you can. After several days, watch how some of the seeds sprout.

If, for whatever reason, your seeds don't sprout, practice nonjudgment—don't get down on yourself and take the outcome personally. Also, practice beginner's mind—with an attitude of curiosity, experiment with less or more water, move the pot to a different location, or add more seeds. As you care for your little plant, your plant cares for you.

Loving-Kindness

Adding a loving-kindness meditation to your formal practice helps to strengthen and clarify intentions, as loving-kindness is a practice of intentions of well-wishing. When you say harmful things to yourself or when someone does something you don't like, the inclination is to judge and be critical of yourself or others. Because infertility has a way of diminishing self-worth and increasing isolation, anger, guilt, and despair, we forget our loveliness. Engaging in practices that help to rewire the brain away from negativity bias and strengthen the "tend and befriend" response is not only important but also essential.

In the tradition of loving-kindness, you repeat four phrases, "May _____ be safe from harm, be healthy, be happy, and have ease of well-being," to five categories of people: yourself, a dear friend, a neutral person, a difficult person, and all beings.

The practice typically begins by sending loving-kindness to yourself, but because we are often so hard on ourselves, it can be easier to start by sending loving-kindness first to someone you care about. It's difficult to love others without loving yourself, so sending well-wishes to yourself is especially important. You then continue to add one category at a time—when ready. This may take many days or weeks before incorporating all categories into the full meditation practice.

When repeating these phrases, intentions of well-being are internalized with increasing depth. When the mind is not obscured by clinging or grasping, it breaks down the boundaries between self and others. When light is brought into the heart through the power of love, it releases harmful thoughts and alarming emotions.

It's not necessary to continue using the traditional phrases; you can always bring in your own. Please know loving-kindness is both a formal practice and an informal practice. Through the day, wherever you are, connecting with intentions of kindness produces feelings of contentment. To deepen this centuries-old practice, the book *Lovingkindness* (2002) by mindfulness teacher and author Sharon Salzberg is a valuable resource.

Formal Meditation: Loving-Kindness Meditation

The following loving-kindness meditation is based on the teachings of Shaila Catherine, founder and principal teacher at Insight Meditation South Bay (IMSB). When using the guided meditation audio tracks (www.janettimarotta. com/meditations), the first ten-minute practice begins by extending loving-kindness to your dear friend and then to yourself. The next ten-minute practice, begins by extending loving-kindness to a neutral person, difficult person, and then all persons everywhere. When practicing without the guided meditation tracks, once you've anchored yourself to your breath, you may wish to send loving-kindness to the first category (yourself or dear friend) and when ready, add each additional category in successive meditations.

Include the following categories:

Yourself. Notice when feelings of loving-kindness arise so you can connect the intentions ever more strongly with the feelings. When sending intentions of well-wishes, it's helpful to visualize the recipient. In this category, place an image of yourself in your *mind's eye*. When you wish well on yourself, you are reminded of being whole and complete as you are and that you are worthy of giving and receiving love.

Dear friend category. Choose a friend, family member, or teacher (someone currently alive and human, whom you are not attracted to) who is basically good. This includes someone for whom you feel positive regard and respect, who is honorable and virtuous.

Neutral person. Choose someone with whom you have no particular involvement or affection toward. This can be anyone, such as the mail deliverer or a grocery clerk. The challenge here is visualizing and sustaining a neutral person in the mind, as the mind is inclined to wander more easily when you have little personal connection or attachment.

Difficult person. Choose someone you are having difficulty with (but not divorcing or being abused by). This category is included because it protects the mind from developing hatred. Negativity is diffused with well-wishes. Loving-kindness is a path of liberation, as it dissolves ill will, which is an obvious enemy. Aversion is weaker than loving-kindness. Love is stronger than hate.

All beings. This category includes all beings throughout the globe. Extending loving-kindness without boundaries expands the heart.

For each category, repeat the four phrases, internalizing the intentions ever more deeply:

- "May _____ be safe."
- "May _____ be healthy."
- "May _____ be happy."
- "May _____ have ease of well-being."

Consider using your own sayings, such as the following:

- "May I trust myself and the qualities I am cultivating to shape my path."
- "May I take good care of my fertile health."
- "May infertility not overshadow my life, and may I take pleasure in what I have."
- "May I recognize my strengths and honor my journey."

When saying the phrases, sense if there's joy arising and say each intention with the wish to be free of suffering. Lift the corners of your mouth into a *half smile* or *Buddha smile,* as this lifts the heart! Coordinating the breath with the phrases is calming, but because loving-kindness is a practice of intentions, your central focus is on the intentions of well-wishes as you are also mindfully breathing. Notice if opposite feelings to loving-kindness arise (e.g., anger, sadness, resentment); these are feelings in the heart being released. You can return to the breath to calm and center or stay with these feelings and bring loving-kindness toward them.

Use the practice log to strengthen and deepen your loving-kindness practice.

Informal Practice: Cultivating Loving-Kindness

Bring loving-kindness into your everyday life—toward those you come into contact with or may be thinking about. When you do a good, honorable human act (such as opening the door for someone, complimenting, helping, or demonstrating concern), notice the qualities you value in yourself. Recognize your inherent goodness and absorb these qualities into your heart. Notice how sending intentions of well-wishes affects your emotional state. Record your experience in the practice log.

Practice Log 7: Formal Practice—Loving-kindness

What did you learn/how did you benefit?   What were your challenges/what interfered?

DAY 1

DAY 2

DAY 3

DAY 4

DAY 5

DAY 6

DAY 7

Practice Log 7: Informal Practice—Cultivating Loving-kindness
Note the influence of bringing loving-kindness towards others.
DAY 1
DAY 2
DAY 3
DAY 4
DAY 5
DAY 6
DAY 7

Eight

FINDING BALANCE IN RELATIONSHIPS

*If we learn to open our hearts, anyone, including the
people who drive us crazy, can be our teacher.*

—PEMA CHODRON

Infertility feels like a life-or-death situation, because in fact it is. When we are unable to bring life into the world or when life is ended prematurely in the womb, infertility is indeed about life and about death. Every area of life is impacted, and the couple's relationship is no different. In the book *Infertility and Identity*, Deveraux and Hammerman (1998, 63–78) explain that when the assumption of having children is challenged, an inalienable right feels denied and men and women's self-esteem is rocked at the core. Because our cultural conditioning links manliness with virility and womanhood with motherhood, infertility is not viewed as a medical condition but rather a personal failure. When self-esteem is threatened to such a primal degree, gender-specific roles become the default mode. But because gender roles are so different, it is difficult for men and women to understand and appreciate how each is coping. Though couples start their relationships on the same team, they now find themselves on opposing sides.

Crisis as Opportunity

When deeply upset at your partner, do you find yourself at the mercy of moods, vulnerable like a shallow-rooted tree in a wild storm? Do you become so disturbed that thoughts go wild, feelings are hurt, and actions become twisted?

When intimately sharing life with another, we come face-to-face with our own reflection, as the life crisis of infertility inevitably drives unresolved issues to the surface. Relationships provide the ultimate arena to wrestle with your most difficult challenges and consequently offer your greatest opportunity for growth.

In Bali, the villager who has suffered the deepest loss within the year is called upon to become the village's high priest or priestess. The Balinese believe the greater the loss, the greater the potential to touch the divine. "Crisis is opportunity" is an expression found in Chinese wisdom. From the West comes the saying "A day without pain is a day without gain."

Mindfulness cultivates the quality of equanimity: the spaciousness of a still and balanced mind, the ability to weather life's ups and downs. Equanimity can also be understood as nonjudgmental openness. It frees the mind from dualistic thinking, where good and bad swings you relentlessly from one side to the other. With a composed mind, it is possible to learn from the wisdom of the paradox: "Your worst enemy is your greatest teacher."

When you inquire within, is the life crisis of infertility an unfair punishment or hidden opportunity?

Understanding Differences

Typically, the very thing that initially drew partners to one another eventually becomes the nemesis of the relationship. That self-possessed, independent quality you so admired in your husband is now accentuated by this crisis, and he now appears cold and shut down. That warm, caring, compassionate quality you so appreciated in your wife is now magnified, and she now appears needy and whiny.

When self-esteem is threatened, gender-specific roles tend to go on automatic pilot: men *fix*, women *engage*. The overfocus on solutions causes men to constrict their emotions, while the overfocus on problems leads women to be overwhelmed by their emotions. Because attempts to fix are ineffective, men often feel inadequate and misunderstood. Conversely, because communication does not yield a sense of connection, women often feel sad and burdened. These competing roles carry a sense of shared loneliness. Not only is there grief about infertility but also a feeling of loss over the emotional relationship and feared loss of a failed relationship all together (Deveraux and Hammerman 1998, 68).

Beyond affecting the emotional realm, infertility affects the sexual arena as well. Because sex and reproduction are intimately tied, the sexual encounter becomes linked with failure and loss. It can feel threatening to become too emotionally close, as letting down your guard can promote feelings of vulnerability.

It may take months or years to become pregnant, either naturally or through pursuing fertility treatment. The longer one tries to become pregnant, the greater the sense of urgency. Increased time brings decreased options and less emotional reserve. This stress carries pressure and frustration into the sexual relationship.

Sex is no longer private and personal once fertility treatment is sought. Sexuality becomes mechanized and scrutinized, significantly impacting intimate bonding. Injections, procedures, monitoring, and surgeries are invasive procedures; hormones are medically stimulated; and fertilization via IVF is achieved outside the body.

When a man and woman share the impact of infertility on their relationship, what does each say? What challenging issues and dynamics in the relationship are identified, and what possibilities are proposed? Here is a summary from the hundreds of men and women with whom I have worked. This definitely resonates with most of the issues and dynamics my husband and I experienced during our own challenge with fertility.

CHALLENGING ISSUES AND DYNAMICS FROM THE MALE PERSPECTIVE

A man often feels confused about knowing how to support his partner. He typically has difficulty understanding what his partner is experiencing, knowing where the boundaries are (leave alone or stay near), and being honest, because his perspective is different and he might say the *wrong thing*. This leads to frustration because good intentions backfire: "I'm damned if I do and damned if I don't."

A common dilemma is: "should I be the *stoic rock* or *sympathetic partner?*" The typical conclusion is: "someone needs to keep an even keel—someone needs to be the *Rock of Gibraltar*, and that someone is me!" But this approach often fails, contributing to distance and disconnection in the relationship.

Because a man often feels the need to be "the protector," he subdues his reaction to a failed IVF cycle or miscarriage, hoping to lessen his partner's added pressures or disappointments. This approach also boomerangs, as his partner tends to perceive him as insensitive and not committed to having a baby. The unfortunate result is that he feels misperceived and undervalued.

A man regularly suffers from seeing his partner suffer—being acutely aware of his partner's distress over others' pregnancies, fears of injections and surgeries, hearing distressing comments, and dealing with complicated situations. A particular concern is seeing his partner take infertility as a personal failure. Because he can do little to remedy the many challenges she experiences, which persist and increase over time, his own feelings of inadequacy consequently stretch and deepen.

It's not uncommon for a man to feel increasingly separated from friends and family, particularly in reaction to his partner's anguish in these circles. He may be aware that others feel like they're on "pins and needles" for fear of saying the "wrong thing" or not knowing how to be supportive. Apart from a few confidants, he typically doesn't talk about infertility to friends or family, compounding a sense of alienation.

The male partner often feels resentful that everything seems to be about infertility: "All resources are going toward building a new house that involves family, while the old house that involves the relationship is being burned down." Having different ideas over family-building options or not having preferences creates further distance.

A man's self-esteem is typically impacted by feeling a diminished role in the sexual relationship. It's not uncommon for him to feel wanted as a sperm donor rather than in an intimate sense. He views his partner as being interested in having sex only when it's linked to pregnancy. Romantic attempts seem to "fall on deaf ears."

Sex often becomes less frequent, spontaneous, or fun. A man generally feels concerned that initiating sex will cause problems, for example, that his partner will feel imposed upon because she is emotionally low or will become sad after sex is over.

It is frequently difficult for a man to integrate work and personal demands—juggling job responsibilities with the requirements of treatment. Common issues of concern include feeling anxiety over not having a family, pressure by his partner's biological clock, concern over the financial costs of treatment, and emotional exhaustion from anticipating treatment results.

CHALLENGING ISSUES AND DYNAMICS FROM THE FEMALE PERSPECTIVE

Because a woman typically tends to focus more on communication issues, she frequently wants her partner to feel more engaged in discussing issues related to fertility. She often perceives herself as giving her all to become pregnant or sustain a pregnancy and views her partner as uninformed and unaware. Disagreements over when to talk about infertility, how much time to converse, and what issues to discuss are habitually met with frustration, adding to a generalized feeling of hopelessness.

A woman often questions whether her partner cares enough, viewing him as "talking the talk, not walking the walk." When her partner focuses on fixing the situation or fixing her emotions, this contributes to not receiving the kind of support needed. She feels judged by her partner when viewed as overreactive or abnormal because she is so overwhelmed by emotions. On the whole, a woman says she feels lonely.

There is an overall expression of frustration or disappointment related to issues of disclosure. It's difficult to reach consensus on how to talk about infertility with others—for example, with whom, when, and how much to disclose. A woman typically complains that her partner wants to disclose to family when she's not comfortable or vice versa. Sometimes, when there is a disclosure agreement, she sees her partner deviating from the plan, which further increases frustration and disappointment.

The impact of infertility on relationships with friends and family is acutely felt by a woman. This includes, for example, hearing the news of someone's pregnancy, being invited to a baby shower, hearing comments experienced as "insensitive," and feeling pressured by family or cultural norms. The repeated bombardment of these events spills over into her intimate relationship.

The overwhelming emotions for a woman are also caused by not knowing how to navigate treatment, how to fit treatment into her already busy life, or how to beat the biological clock. The difficulty of creating a course of action, accessing interpersonal resources, needing infertility to be resolved, or fearing failed outcomes significantly contributes to the stress.

A woman almost universally reports that infertility takes a significant toll on her sexual relationship. A woman who is experiencing infertility routinely has little interest in sex and commonly wonders if the desire to avoid sex is to avoid disappointment, as sex often arouses feelings of sadness and loss. She notes her desire for sex is also decreased by not feeling attractive, being pumped with hormones (which interfere with feeling emotionally OK), balancing sex with work, feeling emotionally exhausted, and having treatment restrictions. Sex often feels like a chore because it is scheduled, mechanized, and oriented around fertility or treatment. It's not uncommon for a woman to want to just "get it over with."

POSSIBILITIES FROM THE MALE PERSPECTIVE

From the male perspective, what helps? With guidance and support, a man often comes to recognize the importance of placing more attention on communication. He recommends expressing his own feelings, starting dialogues, trying to understand his partner's feelings, not trying to *fix* his partner or the situation, letting his partner express, and *listening*. He points to the need for sharing that he has similar feelings even if he doesn't always show his partner and that he communicates in nonverbal ways: "If you want to know how a man feels, watch what he does."

A male partner will come around to suggest placing attention on understanding issues and dynamics, recognizing how big the issue of infertility really is, and realizing he can't *fix* it. He recommends accepting he doesn't react as strongly as his partner and that this is OK: "I don't need to feel guilty, and I am not a bad partner."

The need for self-care is eventually affirmed. Suggestions include exercising, talking with others individually or in a support group, prioritizing important needs, and focusing on stress reduction. The need to work constructively with thoughts, to bring patience and acceptance into the situation, to not put "life on hold," and to think "outside the box" becomes recognized.

To help with loss of control, developing a fertility plan is advocated. This includes exploring family-building options; factoring finances in with emotional costs when making treatment decisions; conveying the importance of parenting over genetics; affirming the potential of parenthood through exploring options; and meeting with others who have pursued adoption, gamete donation, and surrogacy. A man stresses the importance of giving power to their partner in deciding what to do.

Recommendations to enhance the sexual relationship and build intimacy include being more romantic and setting the stage for more intimate encounters. This is achieved by planning activities to create more quality time and by taking greater charge of the social calendar.

When a man is able to hear other women talk about feelings of hopelessness, jealousy, rage, and anxiety, he realizes his partner is not "overreacting." He discovers his partner is not the only one overwhelmed by her emotions, and he reaches a new level of understanding and empathy. This enables him to take his partner's feelings less personally and be more able to *just listen*.

POSSIBILITIES FROM THE FEMALE PERSPECTIVE

What helps from the female perspective? With guidance and support, a woman often comes to suggest broadening her awareness of infertility and understanding the issues and dynamics in her relationship. She points to the need of communicating her fears, concerns, and wishes, having a better sense of what kind of support she needs, asking for what she needs, and even giving her partner a list of support options to choose from. She acknowledges that her partner has a hard time second-guessing a woman's needs and that talking in the car or on walks may make discussion easier. She comes to realize that a lack of emotion in her partner doesn't mean he doesn't care.

A woman will come to emphasize the importance of reducing stress in the relationship by taking an active role in the management of her own well-being. Strategies include reducing stress through mindfulness, joining a fertility group, developing resources, discerning whom to talk with openly, creating a game plan on how to respond to challenging situations, obtaining information on fertility and its treatment, and developing a treatment or adoption plan.

There are various suggestions a woman will make to enhance the sexual relationship, most notably making time to spark sexual intimacy and putting effort into being intimate, because it's important. Ideas include being sexually spontaneous and involved, initiating sex off cycle, separating sex from baby-making time (getting into sex and out of ovulation), reserving a time to be together (e.g., Saturday morning with breakfast in bed), going to bed at the same time as their partner at least a couple of times a week, and even putting sex on a *to do list*—just for fun.

Enhancing the emotional relationship is recognized as also enhancing the sexual relationship. This includes spending more and higher-quality time together, having date nights, being physically intimate, doing little things to get in the mood, broadening the definition of intimacy, texting each other, and traveling to different places, such as going camping or spending the weekend in a bed-and-breakfast.

When a woman hears other men talk about not knowing how to be supportive, she realizes the need to better understand what she herself needs and that it's OK to ask for it. She appreciates that her partner can't mind-read and that asking for her needs to be met in a certain way does not diminish the value of receiving support. She acknowledges her partner isn't able to meet most of her needs and comes to terms with the importance of finding strong support networks outside her relationship, in particular with other women experiencing infertility. When a woman realizes her partner has more feelings than she was aware of and shares deep desires to have children, she is able to feel less hurt, more connected, and better able to reach beyond her relationship for help. Overall, a woman grasps a new understanding—her partner really is upset; he's just not expressing how upset he *really* is!

Where Yin Meets Yang

Men and women's competing gender-specific roles can become complementary by moving toward one another—when men open to their emotions and women focus on solutions. Meeting the opposing forces of infertility with equanimity in one's self and relationship is like finding refuge in the *eye of the hurricane*. It's within these paradoxical twists and turns along the relationship route that navigation is learned and the process guides the direction.

Understanding and working with your partner's different coping style can be both intrapersonally and interpersonally expansive. Rather than each of you representing different parts of the whole, you each become whole and complete on your own. Partners are less threatened when needs are not required to be met by the other. Affirming and adopting coping differences not only help restore balance to the relationship but also enable the issues to be dealt with at a broader and deeper level.

A common stereotype described by John Gray in the best-selling book *Men are from Mars, Women are from Venus* (1992) is that men need to feel sexually connected before they open up emotionally, whereas women need to feel emotionally close before they desire to be sexual. Is this some cosmic joke or ingenious master plan? But this difference can be expansive, as operating outside a stereotypic box fosters growth.

To reclaim sexual intimacy, open to the pleasure of sex, not the goal of pregnancy. Stay *in touch* with one another—hold hands, caress, give one another massages. Prevent your sexual relationship from becoming a medical relationship by keeping your focus on protecting what can only be yours. Diminish the pressure to conceive by focusing on rediscovering sexual attraction, taking breaks from medical treatment, and planning dates. Most importantly, prioritize your relationship. While closeness increases vulnerability, it's vulnerability that leads to courage.

Your relationship presents a wonderful opportunity for practicing mindfulness. When you're with your partner, give your full attention. Make prioritizing the relationship your intention. Create special time together by eliminating interference (e.g., turn your cell phone and laptop off). Participate in activities and time together that foster healing and renewal, such as taking a romantic holiday. Enjoy what you have and what you can do while you don't have children.

Decide when and where to discuss infertility and draw attention to options. Plan how to cope with the holidays—taking a vacation during family holidays may be a great alternative. Focus on gaining information to direct your decisions: *knowledge is power.* Accessing resources through professional support, the Internet, books, and others experiencing infertility helps you take the next step. Each step leads to the next and brings you closer to your child. For some, it's useful to create a plan from start to end point. For others, it's best to just plan one step at a time.

No one wishes to be dealt the infertility card, but when hardship enters uninvited, open to its potential opportunity for growth and move through it as a journey. When couples commit to working on their issues and dynamics, relationships deepen. Being able to find mutual understanding and shared solutions helps grow strength and trust in oneself and each other.

Wise Speech

In Buddhist psychology, our tendency to want to hold on to pleasant feelings, get rid of unpleasant feelings, or choose indifference is called the "three poisons," which are greed (from clinging), hatred (from aversion), and delusion (from indifference). Generally speaking, a woman's tendency to obsess, feel overwhelmed, and personalize experience is an offshoot of clinging, while a man's tendency to dismiss, minimize, turn away, and focus attention elsewhere is an outgrowth of aversion. The tendency toward clinging in one partner and aversion in the other causes couples to feel in opposition and contributes to each feeling misunderstood, blamed, abandoned, or engulfed.

Because relationships are rooted in communication, *wise speech* was considered so important by Buddha that he ranked it as a factor on the Noble Eightfold Path or Path of Awakening. Buddha identified three central components that determine wise speech: *what* you say, *when* you choose to say it, and *whether* it's actually true. When all three factors are simultaneously occurring, you are engaging in wise speech.

Exercise: Paired Listening

The prerequisite to wise speech is being able to *listen—really listen*. Practicing the well-recognized communication exercise called paired listening teaches this first and fundamental step. One partner asks a series of three questions with the intention of just listening, really listening—without needing to say anything back. The other partner has two minutes to answer each question. When completed, roles are reversed. The exercise ends with both sharing the experience with one another. You may choose to ask the questions below or construct your own.

- "Tell me something about how this challenging journey to build a family has impacted your life." (Two minutes.)
- "Tell me something you'd like me to know about you that is important and that you want me to understand." (Two minutes.)
- "Tell me something you love about me." (Two minutes.)
- Reverse (two minutes for each question). Share this experience with one another. (Six minutes.)

It's not uncommon to feel the impulse to speak up, to have an impact in some way. Learning to listen and not interrupt when your partner shares his or her experience of infertility allows you to deal with difficulty in a way that is different from your own. Agreeing or disagreeing is not the point. By listening deeply, you are legitimizing each other's feelings by acknowledging that this is how you're each feeling.

Exercise: Active Listening

A following practice to paired listening is the well-recognized communication exercise called active listening. In this exercise, you tell your partner something you want him or her to understand about you. Your partner listens and then says what he or she heard, without interpreting or offering advice. If you feel your partner understands some but not all of what you are conveying, acknowledge what you felt was understood and misunderstood. Express your message again with greater clarity.

Your partner listens and then says what he or she heard without defending, correcting, or disputing. If there is still part of the message that your partner does not understand, repeat this process again. Continue this back-and-forth exchange until you feel fully understood. When ready, reverse the process.

Don't worry if it takes many attempts before understanding occurs. This exercise is difficult for most couples, and considerable time is needed before true understanding is reached. Because we are more driven by the need to *be right* than the need to *get along*, this exercise is also challenging, as it places understanding at front and center stage.

Active listening is made easier when communication is clear and concise. It's not uncommon for communication to be too long, vague, and overwhelming for the listener. Also, many speak in extremes with black-and-white statements: "You always do this! You never do that!" It's no wonder your partner defends, checks out, attacks back—doesn't listen! When paired listening and active listening become the natural way of communicating, distress lessens and contentment rises.

What does it feel like to be really listened to? How important is it to be understood? What feelings emerge? Have feelings toward your partner changed? Sense if your heart feels more open.

Informal Practice: Cultivating Wise Speech

Focus your communication on wise speech. Pay careful attention to what you say, when you choose to say it, and whether it's actually true. Notice when you are and when you are not engaging in wise speech and the consequences of each. Record what you learned in the practice log.

Chi Kung

Chi kung, also written Qigong, is a Chinese meditative practice that uses slow, graceful movements and controlled deep breathing. Chi means energy or life force, and kung means cultivation of energy or work. Thus, chi kung is the cultivation of energy or work with one's life force. This practice is believed to promote the circulation of chi energy within the body to enhance overall health. Some speculate the practice is beneficial to health through its stress reduction and exercise. Others believe it is the vibrations or electrical currents that are physically circulated through the channels (meridians) that account for the benefits.

There are hundreds of kinds of chi kung. The practice is found in the curriculum of major universities throughout China. Since 1989, medical chi kung has been officially recognized as a standard medicinal tool in Chinese hospitals. Since 1991, medical chi kung has been part of the Chinese national health plan and is a treatment for almost all medical conditions, including infertility. In particular, teaching correct breathing through the chi kung practice is part of the treatment for infertility.

Chi kung is practiced in the United States, included in some stress-reduction programs, and sometimes added as a complementary practice for the treatment of infertility. Chi kung is included here because attuning to the body and increasing energy or life force is so important. It can help to cultivate equanimity and balance in yourself and your relationship.

As an energy practice, chi kung recognizes that the universe is made up of energy and opens your awareness to energy that might otherwise not be noticed. In the practice, energy is sensed in the form of vibrations inside and outside the body. Whether energy is felt or not, the slow, graceful movements and controlled breathing make this another meditation in movement practice.

Formal Practice: Chi Kung

The following sequence is composed of five basic chi kung movements and is also taught by mindfulness teacher and author Bob Stahl in his MBSR classes (www.mindfulnessprograms.com). When using the guided meditation audio tracks (www.janettimarotta.com/meditations), the movements are divided into two ten-minute practices which can be performed separately or back-to-back. You begin by standing in Mountain pose. As you go deeper and deeper into each move, feel the field of energy in and around your body. Record your practice in the practice log.

1. MOUNTAIN POSE

- Stand upright with your eyes closed, feet slightly apart, and weight distributed evenly on your hips. Bend your knees slightly and place your arms to your sides with palms out and chest open. Place your chin parallel to the floor, release shoulders, and straighten the back of your pelvis.
- Stand firm and upright as a mountain—breathing.

2. TAI CHI TWIST

- From Mountain pose, twist to the right, picking up your right toe as your right hand slaps your lower back and your left hand slaps your hip. Reverse directions: twist to the left, picking up your left toe as your left hand slaps your lower back and your right hand slaps your hip.
- Pick up momentum, swinging to the right and left with rhythm, tapping more fully, waking the chi energy in the body, and breathing deeply and fully.

3. Chi Rising, Expanding, Collecting

- From Mountain pose, as you inhale, raise your arms straight out in front as high as your waist with knees bent (energy rising from the palms of your hands).
- Inhale further—spread your arms out wide like a bird, with knees bent (energy expanding from the palms of your hands).
- Exhale—lower your arms down to your sides and straighten your legs (collecting energy into your body).
- Repeat a few more times in a rhythmic flow, feeling the chi energy rising, expanding, and collecting.

4. Chi Ball

- From Mountain pose, rub your palms together rapidly, accumulating chi energy in the form of heat. When sufficiently hot, slowly spread your palms apart as far as the felt field of energy while holding on to the ball of energy or chi ball.
- Shift your weight onto your right foot as you move toward the right, slowly turning the chi ball, so that once to the far right, your right hand is on the bottom and your left hand is on the top.
- Begin to shift your weight off your right foot as you move toward the left, slowly turning the chi ball, so when in front of the body, your hands hold the sides of the chi ball and your weight is equally balanced on both feet.
- Shift your weight onto your left foot as you move toward the left, slowly turning the chi ball, so that once to the far left, your left hand is on the bottom and your right hand is on the top.
- Begin to shift your weight off your left foot as you move toward the right, slowly turning the chi ball, so when in front of the body, your hands hold the sides of the chi ball and your weight is equally balanced on both feet.

- Movement continues, fluidly flowing from right to left, moving the chi ball in the shape of infinity or a sideways number eight.
- Stand in Mountain pose holding on to the sides of the chi ball. Slowly spread your palms, so the chi ball floats to the sky. Feel particles of energy drifting down, permeating your body.

5. KELP FOREST

- As you stand in Mountain pose, visualize yourself as a giant kelp in a magnificent kelp forest. Imagine your feet as the base of the kelp, rooted into the ocean floor; your body as the long, pliable kelp trunk; your arms and hands as the kelp stems and leaves lying to the sides; and your head as the top leaf, which reaches the ocean's surface. Stand tall and motionless in the stillness of the vast ocean.
- As the ocean current begins to pull and waves start to form on the surface, your supple seaweed body undulates with the movement of the aqueous substance in which it's surrounded.
- While the ocean current builds and waves crest on the surface, your seaweed body bends and twists, your seaweed-leaf arms stretch and turn, and your seaweed-top head rolls and falls as you dance in the movement of the ocean. The sun streams down to infuse you and the kelp forest in glistening rays. Sense the energy around you and within you.
- As the ocean now begins to calm, your seaweed body slows its movement, and when the ocean has returned to complete stillness, you stand tall and supple in its tranquility. Soak in the calming energy around and within you.

Practice Log 8: Formal Practice—Chi kung
What did you learn/how did you benefit?   What were your challenges/what interfered?

DAY 1

DAY 2

DAY 3

DAY 4

DAY 5

DAY 6

DAY 7

Practice Log 8: Informal Practice—Cultivating Wise Speech

Note the influence of when you are and are not engaging in wise speech.

DAY 1

DAY 2

DAY 3

DAY 4

DAY 5

DAY 6

DAY 7

Nine

OPENING TO FAMILY-BUILDING OPTIONS

*To understand the heart and the mind of a person, look not
at what he has already achieved, but at what he aspires to.*

—KAHLIL GIBRAN

When the dream of conceiving and carrying a genetically connected child
seems unlikely, a painful juncture is reached. You must choose whether to
do one of the following: (1) end treatment and pursue adoption; (2) continue
treatment using donor eggs, donor sperm, donor embryos, or surrogacy; (3) and
pursue a child-free life or stop with the number of children you already have (secondary
infertility). Struggling with the decision is normal, and honoring the loss
is necessary, for until you've grieved the "loss of the dream," you can't be open to
possibility and discover which route is right for you. What is required next takes
tremendous soul-searching into *who* you are and *what* is truly important.

The decision to pursue your family-building option is a joint venture between
the rational and emotional: weighing your pros and cons, risks and

benefits, treatment analysis, finances, resources, and time, along with what intuitively feels "right" based on your beliefs, upbringing, culture, and needs.

When nearing the end of treatment, you are dealing with two demands that seem worlds apart yet inseparably linked: letting go and turning toward. It's only when you have not given up on but set yourself free from your dedicated course that you can go deeper within the source of your pain to uncover your heart's desire. At this point, when you're at this transitional juncture, vulnerability is the predominant emotion. How could it be otherwise? You are required to move forward when you are nearing the end of a course that has exhausted most of your emotional and possibly financial reserve.

Yet, paradoxically, this time of vulnerability is also a time of immense courage. In daring to venture into third-party parenting, you emerge as a "pioneering parent"—charting a course from the known into the unknown, with a coping strategy built on trust rather than fear and awareness rather than control. You can only choose third-party parenting by moving from your heart.

Loving the Questions

Mindfulness creates a sense of spaciousness, so the mind can be open and able to contain all things without limitation. Mindfulness is met with an attitude of curiosity, as experiencing life without judgment opens the venue to exploration and discovery of one's deeper self. This spacious and curious mind cultivates the quality of patience or understanding that some situations unfold in their own time, without forcing things to be otherwise. You begin to understand it's not the goal but the process that matters, and it's the questions not the answers that are most important.

When choosing to do something unfamiliar, fear is a natural reaction, as the territory of exploration lies outside the comfort zone. When needing to let go of the genetic or gestational tie, it's a nearly universal experience to come face-to-face with your darkest fears. You might find yourself imagining you'll never be able to bond with the child, regretting not having pursued additional treatment, conceiving a child after already having a nongenetically related child, viewing others' genes or prenatal environment as inferior to your own, or believing no option will successfully lead to a child.

You might also fear the child will not be able to bond to you, having issues with identity and self-esteem; being rejected, ostracized, or stigmatized from peers and others; not being fully included in the family lineage; having feelings of frustration due to little or no information about his or her genetic relation; or having emotional, physical, or medical problems.

But all too often, these fears are based on assumptions and erroneous beliefs founded on poor understanding. Mindfulness teaches to apply neutral attention, so your internal experience and external situation do not collide with each other. By taking an informational stance with a willingness to be educated, you can recognize your fears as not necessarily legitimate and access help to identify red flags, determine the best option, and manifest your dream.

Once you've shifted from *needing to be pregnant* to *wanting to parent*, you're ready to pursue third-party parenting. As you shift from a position of fear to trust, you recognize the third-party option not as a failure but as an opportunity.

Understanding the differences, challenges, and benefits among adoption, gamete donation, and surrogacy are essential in choosing the family-building option best for you. Each is explained below, and definitions of third-party parenting terms are given in the appendix under "Fertility 101."

The World of Adoption

There are three types of adoption: domestic, international, and foster-to-adoption, or fost-adopt. This overview includes options, challenges, and benefits for each.

DOMESTIC ADOPTION
The world of domestic adoption has profoundly changed over the last two to three decades. Historically, American adoptions were closed (hidden) and

burdened with secrecy, shame, and denial. Birth mothers were kept out of sight from society, the adoptive parents, and the children. Birth mothers received little support for giving up their babies and were left traumatized. Adoptive parents feared the birth mothers would show up unannounced. Because secrecy implies shame, children who learned of their adoptions later in life by mistake felt betrayed and suffered issues of identity.

In American society today, domestic adoptions are open (exposed), inclusive, and positively viewed. The birth mother and intended parents often develop a relationship during the pregnancy, which continues for a short period past birth. Rather than being a threat, the birth mother is a recognized branch of the family tree.

This open relationship allows the child to feel loved rather than abandoned. While the birth mother may initially have close involvement with the adoptive family, her own life moves on, and contact naturally diminishes over time.

Options for domestic adoption

- Agency versus independent through a private attorney.

Challenges

- Going public, verbally and in print, and waiting for a birth mother to select you.
- Meeting the birth mother and developing a relationship with her and perhaps her family.
- Being able to recognize the "red-flag" issues, such as potential genetic concerns, prenatal exposure to alcohol or drugs, or risky matching issues.

Benefits

- Adopting a newborn.
- Knowing the birth mother, some medical history, and prenatal care.

- Raising a child who may culturally and racially match with your emerging family.

INTERNATIONAL ADOPTION

If you are receptive to adopting a child outside the United States, international adoption agencies specialize in different countries throughout the world. To help children feel connected to their roots and encourage camaraderie among adoptive parents, agencies offer social opportunities for families with children from the same country to connect with one another. Although the child may never know the identity of his or her birth mother, international adoption is open, meaning everyone is aware of the adoption and this knowledge is embraced.

Options for international adoption

- Different countries in many parts of the world.

Challenges

- Completing considerable paperwork, waiting until you're next in line to be matched, and countries closing adoption to the United States without notice.
- Rarely meeting the birth mother and only knowing the genetic and prenatal environment from incomplete written information.
- Accepting a child who is a few months to several years old with potential known and unknown challenges (such as attachment issues, physical abnormalities, or prenatal exposure to alcohol or drugs).

Benefits

- Celebrating multicultural differences.
- Engaging in a humanitarian gesture by providing a home to a child who would not otherwise have one.
- Enabling the child to develop a sense of connection to their country of origin (not to the birth mother who remains unknown).

Fost-Adopt

Children in foster placement or orphanages are waiting to be adopted. If you are open to adopting a child of any age or able to adopt a child who may have physical, mental, or emotional challenges, fost-adopt offers the gift of family to a child in need.

Options for fost-adopt

- Special needs or special circumstances (history of foster homes or orphanages).

Challenges

- Accepting an older child or one who may have emotional or physical challenges.

Benefits

- Engaging in a humanitarian gesture by providing a stable home to a child who does not have one.

Adoption Services

The National Council for Adoption, Creating a Family, and RESOLVE are but a few national infertility and adoption education nonprofits that provide information and support to those interested in adoption. Seek reputable agencies and attorneys who specialize in the kind of adoption best for you. For more personal assistance, adoption consultants bring understanding to the process and help you choose your adoption path. Services often include consultations, support groups, workshops, and referrals to reputable agencies.

Once you're engaged in the adoption process, adoption facilitators can be hired in addition to the agency or attorney to help you personally navigate the process and identify potential red-flag issues. Because the profession is not overseen by a licensure board, screen the facilitator's track record regarding number of years specializing, number of cases completed, and absence of legal issues or complaints. Personal recommendations are always a plus.

The Possibilities of Gamete Donation

The three types of gamete donation include sperm donation, egg donation, and embryo donation. Each is summarized below, and each summary concludes with a review of the challenges and benefits.

SPERM DONATION

The use of donor sperm as a family-building option predates egg donation and embryo donation because medical intervention is not complicated and a home procedure referred to as the "turkey baster method" is possible. In this method, sperm from a known donor (family member or friend) is inserted into the vagina from a needleless syringe or, more recently, from a cup similar to a diaphragm placed in the vagina. However, this option is not recommended, as it is fraught with legal implications, interpersonal complications, and health concerns.

The easiest medical treatment with donor sperm uses *sperm washing* to enhance motility and boost success. This treatment is known as artificial insemination (AI) or interuterine insemination (IUI). This brief and fairly painless office procedure injects sperm into the vagina (AI) through a needleless syringe or into the uterus (IUI) from a thin, pliable tube. When medically necessary, donor sperm is also used in IVF cycles.

Sperm banks are plentiful throughout the United States, and selection of donors is considerable. Regulations related to storage, handling, and screening provide health and legal safeguards, which include quarantining sperm for six months to assure protection from infectious disease. Donor profiles include information on personal and family medical and mental-health history, education, occupation, interests, accomplishments, lifestyle behavior, and motivation. Donors can be excluded on the basis of medical (personal and family), mental, and legal problems. For an additional cost, many sperm banks provide more in-depth information, such as taped donor interviews.

Some sperm banks offer the option to match nonanonymously, enabling intended parents to secure the match once they have personally met the donor. "Identity release" anonymous donors are donors who are willing to meet with the intended parent(s) before donation or after the child is born or with the child after he or she turns eighteen. There are also sperm banks that cater to the lesbian community that include gay donors. Regardless, once the donor is selected, vials of sperm are shipped directly to the clinic of choice to be used in treatment cycles.

An increasing number of donors opt to be on the donor registry. Donors agree to keep their contact information current with the cryobank (sperm bank), which enables the child to contact them once he or she turns eighteen. Approximately 50 percent of children are curious and want to put a face to their donors; thus, this is recognized as a worthwhile option. Once the child meets the donor, there is rarely the need for future contact, as the curiosity need has been met. After the child is born, parents have the option of listing him or her on the sibling registry. Children conceived by the same donor are identified.

To determine readiness to meet the issues and implications of third-party parenting, fertility clinics require intended parents to meet with a therapist who specializes in fertility. The following issues are discussed:

- *Medical.* Understanding the IUI and IVF medical procedures and potential related issues, such as disposition of embryos, number of embryos to transfer, selective reduction, genetic abortion, CCS, and ICSI.
- *Emotional.* Grieving the loss of genetic tie, recognizing the importance of parenting over genetics, acceptance of partially genetically related siblings (secondary infertility) and shared genetics with one parent but not the other, and grappling with the pros and cons of disclosure.
- *Matching.* Being informed of donor agency or donor program options and determining donor selection criteria (such as anonymous versus nonanonymous, donor registry, and characteristics).
- *Legal and financial.* Understanding the need for legal agreement and financial costs.

EGG DONATION

Shortly after the advent of IVF, donor egg became an option. This presents the opportunity for a woman with diminished ovarian reserve (DOR) to experience pregnancy. While DOR most commonly occurs in women thirty-five years and older, it can be a diagnosis for younger women as well. A simple blood test to determine the level of anti-Mullerian hormone (AMH) or follicle stimulating hormone (FSH) tests ovarian reserve, which reflects the size of the remaining egg supply. For women under age thirty-five, a normal AMH ranges from 1.5 to 4.0 nanograms per milliliter. A normal FSH level tested on day three of the cycle is below ten—the higher the number, the closer to menopause.

With a reported 60–80 percent success rate in many clinics, women's odds of success shift in their favor when pursuing donor IVF versus IVF. With equal success rates between fresh and frozen embryos, if the first embryo transfer is unsuccessful, there are often several frozen embryos to transfer for future attempts. Frozen cycles cost significantly less, require less time on medication than fresh cycles, and entail a simple transfer procedure (similar to IUI). Because eggs are often from young women in their early twenties, typical cycles include a substantial quantity of high-quality embryos. Younger eggs also reduce the chance of genetic defects and miscarriage.

Most reputable clinics recommend single embryo transfer (SET) over the previous recommendation of double embryo transfer (DET). It was determined that DET resulted in an average twin pregnancy rate of 20–40 percent. Twin pregnancies are automatically considered high risk, as they have an increased chance of premature delivery and potential long-term health consequences for the babies. Research has concluded the cumulative pregnancy rate for SET is equal to DET. Though SET lowers the probability of pregnancy per cycle, it increases the chances of a healthy child, which needs to be the primary goal.

There is an abundance of egg donor agencies, especially in California, with some agencies specializing in particular races or ethnicities and some donor programs integrated into a fertility clinic. A common disadvantage of a donor program in a fertility clinic is that the donor pool is typically smaller, but it does offer several advantages. These include the following: (1) donors reside within the clinic's geographic area, reducing cost and complexity (air transportation, lodging, coordination); (2) donor program coordinators can facilitate the matching decision because they have met with both the donors and intended parents; (3) and for repeat donors, physicians are able to tailor the protocol on information gained from previous cycles.

Obtaining donor eggs through an egg bank is a fairly recent option, and the success rate between frozen eggs and frozen embryos is almost comparable. Donors are recruited by the egg bank, and eggs from an IVF cycle are retrieved and frozen and can then be purchased in a batch (typically five to eight eggs). The cost of working with an egg bank versus a donor egg agency is lower, and the process is easier and faster. However, there is no guarantee how many eggs will become embryos (best to choose a donor with data on how many previous eggs became embryos or resulted in a pregnancy), and if you match with a repeat donor through an agency whose cycles have resulted in a high number of quality embryos, you have access to all eggs from your paid cycle.

The cost of donor IVF via an agency is typically $30,000 or more. This includes donor, agency, legal, and medical costs (including medical, psychological, and genetic screening of the donor). If you have insurance that covers or partially covers fertility treatment, it does not include donor-specific costs. However, your portion of the IVF cycle (e.g., embryo transfer) may be a covered cost.

When egg donation was initially introduced, about 50 percent of all matches were nonanonymous—donors and intended parents met each other before the match and during the cycle. While most agencies and donor programs today only offer anonymous matching and most donors and intended parents prefer this, there is a recent trend toward "identity release" anonymous donors.

The screening for egg donors is more demanding than it is for sperm donors, because of the medical requirements of the procedure. Egg donors are screened for motivation beyond financial remuneration, ability to reliably participate in the donor cycle, having a lifestyle without excess stress, understanding the medical requirements and potential risks, and not over-identifying with the eggs.

Most intended parents base their matching criteria on the following: race or ethnicity, physical and personality characteristics, personal and family medical-health background, education, intelligence, interests, lifestyle behaviors, and "intuitive feel."

The American Society of Reproductive Medicine (ASRM) provides screening guidelines for donors to which all reputable clinics adhere. Guidelines include the need for medical, genetic, and psychological screening with a licensed clinician who specializes in fertility. The psychological evaluation includes a one-hour interview and a personality profile (Personality Assessment Inventory (PAI) or Minnesota Multiphasic Personality Inventory (MMPI)), which screens for psychopathology. These profiles also include validity scales, which determine if the donor applicant reliably portrays herself.

When egg donors are family members or friends, they are referred to as known donors. Having a sister as your donor maintains a genetic connection to the family, as sisters share 50 percent genetics. Known donors (egg and sperm) and surrogates are considered to be the *best and worst* matches: These arrangements are best when the relationship is void of unresolved issues (e.g., sibling rivalry), open disclosure is comfortable and agreed upon, and the family is supportive. Otherwise, family holidays and get-togethers can be awkward and strained, and relationships can become difficult to manage. Known donations cultivate generosity for the donor, gratitude for the intended parents, and a life-affirming personal transaction for all.

ASRM also includes screening guidelines for intended parents using egg donation. Similar to sperm donation, the psychological consultation focuses on *readiness* to address the issues and implications of egg donation, such as issues of disclosure; loss of the genetic tie; and awareness of the medical, financial, and legal issues. A personality inventory is not required.

Embryos from an egg bank or donor agency are often frozen before transfer, and thus no cycle coordination between the donor and intended parent (recipient) is necessary. However, in the case of an agency donor, cycle coordination is necessary if the clinic recommends transfer of an embryo from a fresh cycle.

EMBRYO DONATION

The success rate, particularly for donor IVF, is so high that it can result in extra stored frozen embryos that are not needed once a family feels complete. Most individuals or couples pay the annual storage fee ($700 or more) for one or more years, and then they need to act on their decision regarding disposition of extra embryos. Their options include disposing, donating to science, or donating to an individual or couple in need. Though most select the first two options, an increasing number of parents are choosing to donate their embryos to others who also struggle with infertility.

Some fertility centers have an embryo donor program, which consists of embryos from IVF, donor egg IVF, or donor egg or sperm IVF cycles. The individual or couple donating embryos and the intended parent(s) or IP(s) independently meet with a fertility counselor to determine readiness in dealing with the issues and implications of embryo donation. A personality inventory is not required. While the advantages of embryo donation over egg donation include reduced cost and minor medical intervention, the disadvantage is reduced selection on matching criteria. Embryo donation is a particularly good choice for single women who need both a sperm and egg donor. For those who wish to meet the embryo donors, Christian-based agencies help in the matching process and treat the donation as an adoption.

DONOR GAMETE CHALLENGES AND BENEFITS

Challenges

- Imbalance or absence of genetic connection to IP(s).
- Concern over issues of disclosure to child and others.
- Genetically related siblings from the same donor (in particular, donor sperm).
- Fear of failed outcome.
- Financial considerations.

Benefits

- Ability to carry a pregnancy.
- Control over lifestyle choices that can impact pregnancy.
- An intentional birth.
- Substantial donor information, choice, and healthy genetic background.

The Heart of Surrogacy

Couples often come to surrogacy as a last resort, hoping simply to survive it. However, this path to parenthood, with its intimate transaction of life and hope, will often transform both surrogate and recipient. Surrogacy is a journey; as with all journeys, it offers much more than a trip from point *A* to point *B*. Surrogacy can put you on a "heart's path," transforming your view of self, the world, and your child.

THE MATCH

The single most important factor in the surrogacy experience is the relationship between you and your surrogate. This is where you create a legacy for your child. Nurturing this relationship promotes the genuine exchange of love and trust found at the core of this process. In this way, the three of you create a child born out of generosity and compassion.

The foundation for a surrogacy birth rests on personal compatibility between you and your surrogate. Out of this relationship, a child will be born, grow, and develop part of his or her identity. Good matches begin with honest self-appraisals. Surrogacy is an intimate experience and makes heavy demands upon trust. You begin this process by sharing how each of you views the complexities of surrogacy and how you have dealt with other challenges in your lives.

While often challenging, the relationship with your surrogate can be truly transformational. When you let go of control and allow another woman into your relationship to carry your child, your ego's clutch loosens. It is difficult to let go of that part of you that seeks identity and personal satisfaction by possessing what is yours. Much can happen when this door is opened, and much that happens depends on the individual. Surrogacy demands that you accept having no control over this aspect of life and places you in the arms of humanity and into the womb of another woman.

When you "dare to be different" and have your child in a way that doesn't match your dreams and societal norms, you enter an arena that appears threatening. You stretch beyond your comfort zone. You have no choice but to expand.

THE SURROGACY RELATIONSHIP

What is important about the relationship with your surrogate is not how close you are to one another but how genuine you are with one another. You must respect the agreements set forth from the beginning, accept the differences, and vow to work on difficulties as they arise. The strength of the relationship eases or eradicates your fears and is worth many times the cost of the signed contract.

When you embrace the surrogacy relationship, you become a parent who is proud to have a child born in this way. You can let go of the fear of disclosure to friends, family, and your child. Your child's feelings will match your feelings. If you are enthusiastic about bringing your child into the world in this brave way, your child will feel whole. If you embrace the humanitarian gesture of surrogacy, your child can inherit the world as a generous place.

THE COUPLE'S RELATIONSHIP

While surrogacy can be particularly threatening to your relationship with your partner, it is a challenge that can also deepen your relationship. Seeing another woman enter your intimate territory by carrying your baby can elicit feelings of jealousy, resentment, guilt, and anger. While the surrogate represents your hope for a child, she also represents your loss of a child. No one comes to surrogacy without loss.

While knowing full well that this pregnancy is consciously and mutually planned, negative feelings can nevertheless, at times, take over. These times of crisis can be periods of growth. This is where you learn to attune to the longer rhythms of life and connect with what is "trying to happen." You focus on the meaning or essence of this experience. This is about bringing a child into the world. It is about trust and ultimately about love. Your relationship with your partner can deepen because you are able to connect with what is truly important. Entering into this transaction of love can rekindle your marriage vows and strengthen what you hold sacred in your relationship.

Coming from the Heart

The surrogacy relationship is a journey about how to grieve, how to let go of fear, and how to find acceptance and trust. This relationship can deepen and strengthen who you are as individuals and as a couple. Ultimately, this venture enables you to really understand that a child is an expression of love and comes from the heart.

Surrogacy Options, Types, and Challenges

Options

- Agency, independent (self-advertise—not recommended), or personal (family or friend).

Types of surrogacy (sperm from partner or donor)

- Gestational—egg from intended mother via IVF and embryos transferred to gestational carrier.
- Donor gestational—egg from donor via IVF and embryos transferred to gestational carrier.
- Traditional—egg from surrogate via IUI or Artificial Insemination (not commonly pursued or recommended).

Challenges

- Not employing an agency, which places intended parents at risk due to lack of expertise (e.g., legal contract, medical insurance, payment).

- Making decisions related to agency and surrogate selection.
- Being able to match on issues regarding genetic abortion, selective reduction, amniocentesis, number of embryos to transfer, and degree of closeness.
- Being able to afford surrogacy.
- Managing the surrogate-intended parent relationship.
- Managing personal emotions and couple's issues and dynamics.

Disclosing Birth Rite

Open adoption is now the norm, because closed adoption has shown that secrecy implies shame, and children who accidentally learn of their adoptions feel betrayed. Gamete donation has yet to fully grapple with issues of disclosure. In today's current climate, anonymous matching is the norm, not all intended parents choose disclosure, the majority of donors elect not to be on the donor registry, and the majority of intended parents do not choose their donors based on the donor registry.

As parents of children from adoption, gamete donation, or surrogacy, *what*, *when*, and *how* do you talk to your children about *where* they have come from and *why* they have come to be?

Why? The hesitancy to disclose is based in part on the concern that children will be psychologically wounded in some way. But in an article that summarized the effects and outcomes of third-party reproduction, Greenfeld (2015) states children conceived through third-party reproduction do well psychologically and developmentally, and in another summary article, Zweifel (2015) states parents do well also, but mothers who don't disclose to their children often have higher levels of distress than those mothers who do disclose.

There is no longer dispute over whether to tell your child about his or her genetics and gestation, as the pros for open disclosure far outweigh the cons. In particular, professionals believe that every child has a "right to know" his or her birth story. From the adoption literature, we've learned that accidental disclosure produces a sense of shame and betrayal. In the case of gamete donation, it is possible for the "secret" to be discovered not only through a friend or family member but also through such medical procedures as blood typing or genetic coding. With recent advances in medicine, genetic history is becoming increasingly important and playing a critical role in prevention and treatment. Denying your child the right to this knowledge may impede the access of optimal medical care. But the endorsement of open disclosure applies to the United States and may not be the recommended option in other countries. Cultural factors are significant and need to be weighed into the decision of whether or not to disclose.

Where? In exploring why you want a child, you invariably begin questioning what makes a family and pondering over the relative contribution of genetics versus environment or nature versus nurture. You must ask yourself, "Where does the child come from—the genetic contributor, the gestational carrier, or my heart?" You must confront your fears and believe that you will bond with the child and the child will bond with you; that the genetics or prenatal environment are not inferior or defective; that family, friends, or society will accept the child and not doubt the "real" attachment (and if not, it is their loss or limitation); that your self-worth will be validated; and that a child will someday, somehow come to you.

How? When you've grieved the loss of genetic tie or inability to carry a pregnancy and embraced third-party parenting, the child will mirror your comfort level. If you welcome this path, the child will have little if any issue with loss or identity. Disclosure is an evolving process and needs to match with the child's developmental stages of understanding. Photo albums can serve as worthy introductions. Children's books on being born from ART and third-party parenting are highly recommended, as they teach family comes in different shapes, colors, and sizes.

When? Integrating the knowledge of third-party parenting early, in an age-appropriate way as cognition level matures, can help the child understand and internalize his or her genetic heritage. It is never recommended to tell your child during adolescence, as this is a time teeming with identity issues. Telling your child after adolescence could bring a sense of betrayal, producing an indignant response: "Why are you telling me this now?"

What? What you say should be what you believe and know to be true for you. It reflects what you've discovered in the process and how you've come full circle. Examples include the following:

- "This is someone who helped us have you."
- "You grew from her womb while you grew from our hearts" (surrogacy.)
- "Your family tree has many branches."
- "The more love the better."
- "The world is a generous place."
- "Look what happens when you ask for help."

Gamete donation and surrogacy are becoming increasingly chosen family-building options, and there is no scarcity of books and resources. As starters, you may find benefit in *Mommies, Daddies, Donors, and Surrogates: Answering Tough Questions and Building Strong Families* by Diane Ehrensaft (2005) and *Building a Family with the Assistance of Donor Insemination* by Ken Daniels (2004). The Donor Conception Network at dcnetwork.org is a helpful website that includes information on how to talk about donor conception. "Pioneering parents" give birth to "pioneering children." The legacy these children carry speaks of a profound humanitarian gesture of generosity, trust, and belief in what it means to be part of the human family.

Exercise: Active Listening

When discussing your fertility plan, to help guide your discussion and focus on understanding, practice active listening. As described in chapter 8, one partner answers each question, and the other partner listens and repeats what he or she heard. When the first partner feels fully understood, reverse. Below are some examples of constructive questions:

- "How do you understand our current fertility plan? What are your fears? What are your intentions?"

- "Are you open to pursuing a third-party option if trying naturally or IVF is not successful? What are your fears? What are your intentions?"
- "How will you know when it's time to stop trying to have a child using the way we are trying and time to move on? What are your fears? What are your intentions?"

Smiling with Gratitude

Filling the emotional space created by infertility with gratitude can help you let go and turn toward that which is difficult. A few years ago, my friend's twenty-year-old son passed away in a tragic accident. Being long-time meditators, the parents sought support from their spiritual teacher, who instructed them to hold their profound loss in gratitude. In their son's celebration of life gathering, they stressed how love never dies, how blessed they were to have had him in their lives, and how grateful they were to have this circle of love and support around them. They simultaneously acknowledged their loss while filling their hearts with gratitude. They asked for everyone's support by doing the same.

Thich Nhat Hanh stresses that life is a miracle and how important it is to "count your blessings"—the blue sky, the breath, the tall grass. He reminds us that life is full of pain and beauty and to recognize what's not wrong. "How can I smile when I am filled with such sorrow? It is natural—smile at your sorrow because you are more than your sorrow" (Ryan 2007, 55). Thich Nhat Hanh asserts that when life is going well, it's important to acknowledge what is there to appreciate, but it's even more important to acknowledge what is there to appreciate when life is filled with difficulty. Making concurrent room for suffering and gratitude softens the heart and soothes the soul.

In his book *Thanks: How the New Science of Gratitude Can Make You Happier* (2007), Robert Emmons, the leading researcher on gratitude and happiness, defines gratitude as the "*acknowledgment* of goodness in one's life"—saying "yes" to life—and "*recognizing* that the source(s) of this goodness lie at least partially outside the self—giving thanks to the giver" (2007, 4).

Emmons demonstrates that gratitude has been found to increase happiness, hopefulness, and life satisfaction and to decrease materialistic tendencies and jealousy toward others' success.

Author M. J. Ryan (2009) shows how to fill your life with giving and receiving joy through gratitude and cites studies on the emotional and physical benefits of doing this:

> It seems that when we recognize ourselves and our lives as the precious opportunities they truly are, we take better care of ourselves. It also makes us kinder and more generous to others, less materialistic, more forgiving, more able to deal with stress, and less prone to bitterness, envy, resentment, and greed. When you take all these good effects together, practicing appreciation adds 6.9 years to your life, which is greater statistically than stopping smoking or exercising.

Ryan hypothesizes that when we think positive thoughts such as gratitude, "we are bathing our bodies/minds/spirits in good or bad chemicals based on our thoughts. And gratitude is one of the most powerful positive chemical creators!" (2009, 15–16).

Gratitude leads to generosity and a sense of belonging to our common humanity (Moffitt 2002). Of all the compassion practices, gratitude is the easiest to cultivate and is especially helpful when challenged by fertility. The more you practice gratitude, the more light is available to shine on times of darkness. Gratitude grows strength and courage—flowers grow where thorny bushes would have otherwise multiplied.

Exercise: What's Not Wrong—The Gratitude List

What's not wrong is a mindfulness practice that helps cultivate gratitude. It trains the brain to focus on what's not wrong rather than on what's wrong. A common exercise that steers the brain in this wholesome direction is the "gratitude list." On the top of a sheet of paper, write something you feel grateful for. Each day, add to the list until the sheet is filled from top to bottom. Keep this gratitude list by your bed so you can go to sleep and wake up remembering to count your blessings!

Informal Practice: Cultivating Gratitude

Throughout the day, notice the impact of gratitude on your mood and actions. You may choose to record how gratitude has affected you. For example, when walking down the street and appreciating the green trees or sun on your face, how did you feel and how were your actions affected? Record your informal gratitude practice in the practice log.

Aspiration Meditation

Aspiration practices are used to access the innate healing potential within. In the Buddhist tradition, these practices involve expressing intentions of well-being and a willingness to move closer to what you fear. From a Buddhist perspective, everything you do starts from a place of intention. When combining words or verses into a meditation, you can cross over from where you are in this present moment to where you *intend* to be.

Aspiration practices can be used as a formal or informal practice and be adapted in different ways for any challenge or situation. One possibility is to use the breath to cultivate gratitude. We tend to take the breath and the life that is given to us for granted. This inclination causes feelings of loneliness and separation. Finding gratitude in the breath helps to strengthen the connection to our life source and to all living beings. We feel bonded by our common humanity.

Formal Practice: Aspiration Meditation

To begin, settle into a place of quiet. Bring light attention to the breath, noticing where the breath is most prominent in the body. Feel the rhythmic flow of the breath cycle and ride upon its currents. Raise the corners of the mouth into a half smile. This small upturning of the mouth lifts your heart and lightens your spirit. Sense if there's calm arising. Open your heart to draw in aspirations of gratitude, internalizing these aspirations more deeply with each breath. You can coordinate the phrases with the in-breath and out-breath or simply continue to mindfully breathe as you say each phrase. Choose to repeat these phrases or phrases of your own.

"May I find gratitude in the breath."
"May I find gratitude in each moment."
"May I find gratitude in the qualities I have cultivated."
"May I find gratitude in the love that surrounds me."
"May I find gratitude in the beauty of nature and life itself."

Record this practice in the practice log and note what you learned. Listen to the guided aspiration practice at www.janettimarotta.com/meditations.

Mindful Inquiry: Pregnancy Versus Parenthood

Find a comfortable resting position. Slowly close your eyes and simply notice the breath naturally occurring. As you bring light attention to the breath, invite the breath to slow and deepen on its own. Follow the breath sensations in the body as you're riding on the breath waves, feeling the rhythmic flow.

Drop into your heart and imagine breathing into and out from your heart. On the inhalation, feel the heart opening and expanding. On the exhalation, feel the heart softening and relaxing. Open to this practice of inquiry by asking yourself this question: "Is my true longing pregnancy or parenthood? Do I really need a genetic tie to connect with my child, or can I connect through love?" As your heart opens wide, invite the answers to enter.

Practice Log 9: Formal Practice—Aspiration Meditation

What did you learn/how did you benefit?   What were your challenges/what interfered?

DAY 1

DAY 2

DAY 3

DAY 4

DAY 5

DAY 6

DAY 7

Practice Log 9: Informal Practice—Cultivating Gratitude
Note the influence of gratitude on your mood and actions.
DAY 1
DAY 2
DAY 3
DAY 4
DAY 5
DAY 6
DAY 7

Ten

GIVING BIRTH TO YOURSELF

When the way comes to an end, then change.
Having changed, you pass through.

—I CHING

*H*aving the willingness to venture into the unknown territory of infertility
takes real courage. As Anais Nin says, "Life shrinks or expands in proportion to one's courage." But when your path is built with mindfulness qualities
and you're held in the arms of compassion, how can you not expand and find
what you are looking for?

As you integrate the teachings and practices into your fertility journey,
you develop trust as self-reliance and look within yourself for what is true. You
recognize your whole and complete self is already here. Your original goodness
rises to the surface, and you understand the meaning of Lao Tzu's words: "Be
really whole and all things will come to you."

Nothing Is Everything

Generosity, or giving without needing to get anything in return, is the first practice taught by the Buddha and also considered the highest. It's the most basic act that frees you from the root of suffering—clinging to what you want or resisting what you don't want as though your life depended on it. When you let go of assumptions, expectations, needs, and ideas about how you or your experience craves to be, a sense of spaciousness and ease of well-being emerges. To loosen the grip of craving, you participate in the very practice of letting go—generosity.

To help shift from a position of scarcity to one of abundance, from *me, mine, and I* to interconnectedness, cultivating generosity is a worthy ally. As you learn to change the way you relate to others with compassionate care, you are simultaneously able to relate to yourself with unconditional love. Generosity breaks down the barriers that separate you from others—this enables you to recognize your true nature is whole and complete already.

Informal Practice: Cultivating Generosity

When going about your day, notice how you feel when you have selflessly given. This might be in the form of a kind deed, gift, supportive gesture, or smile. Also notice when you are the recipient of a generous act.

Savor the kindness, goodwill, experience of common humanity, and connection to basic goodness in yourself and others that generosity bestows. Invite the joy to permeate deeply so you can remember to incline the mind toward these feelings of positivity wherever you are. Note your experience in the practice log.

Tonglen

The Tibetan Buddhist "heart practice" called *tonglen* strengthens our capacity to care and connect with ourselves and others. This practice draws from the wisdom of paradox to reverse our tendency to cling to what we want and resist what we don't want. This practice instructs you to *take in* pain by breathing in suffering and to send out relief from suffering by breathing out ease and well-being.

Tonglen cultivates the quality of openness by expanding your ability to feel emotions. Tonglen also cultivates the quality of generosity by releasing unconditional acceptance and compassion for yourself and others. The practice strengthens your capacity to accept the three truths of reality: to reduce resistance to suffering and learn to be with it (*dukkha*—dissatisfaction); to lessen the need for permanence and acknowledge that all things change in time (*anicca*—impermanence); and to decrease attachment to a permanent, separate sense of self and recognize your true nature or original goodness (*anatta*—no self).

The practice shifts perspective from individuality to mutuality, independence to interdependence, and self-centeredness to selflessness. You recognize common humanity and wish for all beings' happiness and well-being.

Tonglen is both a formal and informal practice, with several variations. One version is to breathe in suffering of someone close to you and breathe out release of that suffering. Another form is to breathe in your own suffering and that of others similarly challenged and then breathe out relief and happiness to yourself and others. When you're feeling happy, another form is to breathe in suffering, wishing freedom from suffering for all, and breathe out relief, wishing happiness for all. A wonderful description of tonglen and its different forms is presented by American Buddhist nun Pema Chodron in her book *When Things Fall Apart* (2000, 93–97).

Formal Practice: Tonglen

To begin the practice of tonglen, rest your mind in openness. Breathe into and out from your heart, noticing the heart opening, expanding, relaxing, and softening. Once you have anchored to the breath, grounded to the body, and opened with your heart, with each breath ever so slowly breathe in the heaviness, density, and darkness of the emotional toll of infertility. This may include a sense of anxiety, insecurity, fear, or confusion.

With each increasing in-breath of heaviness, breathe out a feeling of spaciousness, softness, and light. This may include a sense of confidence, wholeness, or calm. With each in-breath, allow the heaviness, density, and darkness of infertility to deepen. With each out-breath, invite the lightness to soften, soothe, and relax.

As you breathe in, slowly expand the pain you take in to include others similarly challenged by fertility. You may begin with someone you hold dear and then include others lesser known. Continue to expand to those who share this challenge in your city, state, country, and finally to the entire world. As you breathe out, send relief, light, and compassion to others.

As you relate as a compassionate being, intimately sense the connection to yourself and others and mutual wish for happiness. Feel this intention of well-being grow stronger, deeper, and more nourishing with each breath. Remember to record your practice on the practice log and to access the guided tonglen practice at www.janettimarotta.com/meditations.

Returning to Your Deep Intention

As you find a comfortable resting position by either lying down on your back or sitting up with a straight spine, slowly close your eyes. Take three deep, long breaths—inhaling through the nostrils and exhaling tension and tightness from the mouth. Return to breathing at your own natural rhythm—inhaling and exhaling from your nostrils. With light attention on the breath, invite the breath to slow and deepen on its own. Feel the breath in the body as you're riding upon the current of each and every breath wave.

Drop into your heart as you imagine breathing into and out from your heart. On the inhalation, feel the heart opening and expanding. On the exhalation, feel the heart softening and relaxing.

Enter into this practice of inquiry by recollecting the original intention that brought you on this mindful fertility journey. Ask yourself, "What is the deep motivation that led me to this book? Have I uncovered my purpose, my wish? What qualities have I cultivated to sustain me on this journey? How can I continue to nurture my intention as I venture forward?"

As your heart opens wide, invite the presence of mind and qualities you've cultivated on this *fertile path* to arise within.

Practice Log 10: Formal Practice—Tonglen

What did you learn/how did you benefit?   What were your challenges/what interfered?

DAY 1

DAY 2

DAY 3

DAY 4

DAY 5

DAY 6

DAY 7

Practice Log 10: Informal Practice--Cultivating Gratitude
Note the influence of selfless giving and being the recipient of a generous act.

DAY 1

DAY 2

DAY 3

DAY 4

DAY 5

DAY 6

DAY 7

Epilogue

Mindfulness shows that meaning is in the journey, wisdom is in the paradox. Infertility is not seen as an obstacle but a challenge, not as a crisis but a hidden opportunity for growth. You cultivate acceptance to be with what is and turn toward that which you resist. Then, and only then, can you break free from suffering and understand the ancient proverb "The way out is the way through."

You notice the habitual tendency to fall into obsessive thoughts of past regret and future fear—floating phantoms of *if only, why me, it's not fair.* You anchor to the present moment and arrive with calm at the doorway of your life. With clarity of vision to think unhampered and qualities cultivated to protect and sustain, you chart your course with a wise mind and open heart.

Seeing through the lens of nonjudgmental awareness shows there's no such thing as success and failure—everything is here for the learning. Fertility treatment doesn't fail when you take the information learned from each attempt to steer your path. The shortest route between *A* and *B* is not necessarily the most direct or best route, when you find what your heart is truly searching for.

You come to know it's not *resolving* infertility but *integrating* it. It's not *in spite of* infertility but *because* of it that your child will come to you. You find strength in knowing that if you stay open to possibility, you will have a child.

During challenging situations with friends or family, when unexpected waves appear off starboard deck, you recognize "your worst enemy is your greatest teacher." When you've met an impasse and don't know whether to go east or west, remember to love the questions, as the questions are more important than the answers. And when you fear the storm will never calm, know nothing is permanent. Gain comfort in the mantra "All things shall pass."

When distressing thoughts like cumulus clouds come your way, the mind like the sky has no limits. Watch these mental formations lose their form and float away. Know that if you make space for emotions and allow grief to unfold, sorrow gives way to compassion, and compassion gives way to gratitude.

Every loss brings you a step closer to your child. Find strength in knowing you'll emerge perhaps with a different understanding of family and stronger than you were before. The gratitude found when you do have a child will make you the parent you would probably not have become.

Rather than concentrating on the results, recognize it's the work itself that matters. If you find yourself wishing you or your situation would change, notice your resistance and stop trying to fix what's broken, for not until you accept yourself as you are, are you free to change. Remember, when you're not trying to change, change naturally occurs. You become the change agent yourself.

When you accept yourself unconditionally, the boundary between *self* and *other* dissolves. As you let go of the assumptions and interpretations that falsely define and confine your sense of self, you are able to see infertility not as a definition of who you are but the medical condition it actually is. You witness the arising of your true nature or original goodness—your whole and complete self, with your varied imperfections and inadequacies. You relinquish the delusion of a separate *self* and recognize you are part of the world and the world is part of you.

In the very quest to bring new life into the world, you bring your whole and complete self as you are with you. When coming from the *outside in*, fertility is outside your reach, but when coming from the *inside out*, fertility is already here.

Infertility is a catastrophe in every sense of the word.
Yet it is the very struggle of infertility and its diminishing of your reserves
in every domain of your life that can ultimately replenish and further you.
It requires you to look for happiness not on the outside but on the inside.
The continual contractions—through withdrawal, resentment, fear, and panic—
make you thirst for expansion: trust, acceptance, peace, and finally liberation.
Everyone seeks happiness,
and it is at this very moment when happiness seems lost
that the human spirit will fight hardest to find happiness where it lives.
The final paradox is that infertility is inevitably a birthing process.
The labor is difficult and frightening, and we resist,
but the process carried through brings forth a new spirit in all who are open to it.

Appendix Fertility 101

Evaluation and Treatment Considerations

HOW LONG SHOULD IT TAKE TO BECOME PREGNANT?

On average, for women age twenty to thirty, there is a 20–25 percent probability of conception per month; between age thirty and thirty-five, probability is 15 percent per month; and over thirty-five, probability is less than 10 percent per month. Fertility typically starts to *dip* at age thirty-five and declines rapidly after forty. Increased age impacts egg quantity and quality and determines the ratio of genetically normal eggs.

HOW LONG SHOULD I WAIT TO SEE A FERTILITY SPECIALIST?

It is generally recommended that women over age thirty try to conceive for six months before seeing a fertility specialist and women under age thirty try to conceive for twelve months before seeing a fertility specialist. However, recent evidence suggests that waiting an additional six months may not add much value. For women with a history of reproductive problems, waiting three to four months is recommended. Go directly to a fertility clinic as opposed to your OB or GYN if you are concerned about your age or how long you have been trying to conceive or if you "sense" there may be an issue.

WHAT IS INCLUDED IN THE MEDICAL EVALUATION FOR FERTILITY?

Tests for men include medical history; semen analysis; possible additional sperm, blood, and cultures tests; and consultations to assess structural problems or blockages. Tests for women include medical history, egg quality analysis, testing of ovulation, examining fallopian tubes and uterus, and checking cervical mucus.

WHAT IS THE COST AND COVERAGE FOR IVF?

The cost for IVF varies across clinics but approximates $20,000 and increases with additional recommended procedures, such as ICSI. Coverage varies across states and insurance plans. Some clinics offer IVF insurance such as ARC Fertility, which includes financing options and shared-risk packages that include partial reimbursement if pregnancy does not occur.

HOW DO YOU CHOOSE AN IVF CLINIC?

Always choose a reputable clinic in good standing with American Society of Reproductive Medicine (ASRM) and with a long track record of using assisted reproductive technology (ART). Though clinic IVF statistics are available on the web, these statistics can be misleading. For example, some clinics have higher patient-selection standards, which skew the data.

Hormones and Testing

HORMONES

- *Estrogen.* A primary female hormone, produced by the ovaries, placenta, and adrenal glands.
- *Testosterone.* The primary male hormone, which influences the production and maturation of sperm.
- *FSH—Follicle Stimulating Hormone.* A hormone (gonadotropin) produced by the pituitary gland that stimulates the growth of the

follicle surrounding an egg. FSH may also be given by injections during IVF.

- *AMH—Anti-Mullerian Hormone.* A hormone produced by granulosa cells in ovarian follicles, which tests ovarian reserve and reflects the size of the remaining egg supply.
- *LH—Luteinizing Hormone.* A hormone produced by the pituitary gland, which normally causes ovulation and eggs to mature.
- *GnRH—Gonadotropin Releasing Hormone.* A hormone produced by the hypothalamus that prompts the pituitary gland to release FSH and LH into the bloodstream.
- *hCG—Human Chorionic Gonadotropin.* A hormone produced by the placenta measured in pregnancy tests. It may also be injected to stimulate ovulation and maturation of eggs.

TESTING

- *BBT—Basal Body Temperature Chart.* Daily charting of temperature to help determine ovulation, performed due to the rise of progesterone after ovulation and the drop at or just before menstruation, when both estrogen and progesterone levels fall.
- *FSH Test.* Blood taken on day three of the menstrual cycle. FSH indicates ovarian reserve—egg viability. The higher the FSH, the less reserve. Levels below ten suggest higher probability of success.
- *HSG—Hysterosalpingogram.* X-ray procedure that determines if the fallopian tubes are open and if there are abnormalities in the uterus.
- *Laparoscopy.* A surgical procedure that may be used for diagnostic evaluation as well as reparative surgery (e.g., endometriosis) and other fertility procedures.
- *Pregnancy Test.* Blood or urine test that determines a clinical pregnancy: confirmed pregnancy = high HCG level, chemical pregnancy = low HCG level, suggesting possibility of pregnancy but requires further testing to confirm.

Fertility Diagnoses

FEMALE FACTOR
When infertility is related to the woman.

MALE FACTOR
When infertility is related to the man.

OHSS—OVARIAN HYPER-STIMULATION SYNDROME
It's a potential risk of IVF due to the ovaries being overstimulated by the hormone injections. Enlargement of the ovaries, fluid retention, and weight gain can result. IVF clinics closely monitor the cycle through ultrasound to avoid what can become a potentially life-threatening risk, albeit extremely small.

ENDOMETRIOSIS
Endometrium grows outside the uterus, resulting in scarring, pain, and heavy bleeding, often damaging fallopian tubes and ovaries.

FIBROID TUMORS
It's a tumor in the uterus, which may prevent implantation or cause miscarriage.

PCOS—POLYCYSTIC OVARY SYNDROME
The most common endocrine disorder in reproductive-age women, with 5–10 percent prevalence. Ovaries contain many small follicles or cysts that may not grow normally and regress before the time of ovulation. There are many possible symptoms; among these are menstrual irregularities and impaired fertility. In women with PCOS, failure to ovulate is the most common reason for not conceiving.

AUTOIMMUNE FACTORS
Immune factors are those that may decrease or impair fertility, such as thyroid disorders and antibodies to sperm—substances in the male or female blood

and in reproductive secretions that reduce fertility by causing sperm to stick together, coating their surfaces, or killing them.

Treatments and Procedures

Intrauterine Insemination (IUI)
It is sometimes referred to as artificial insemination; the sperm is washed free of seminal fluid to increase the chance of fertilization and then inserted directly into the uterus. Clomid and injectables (stimulating hormones) may be added to further enhance fertility.

Assisted Reproductive Technology (ART)
It is advanced medical treatment that involves handling human eggs or embryos. The most recognized treatment is IVF.

In Vitro Fertilization (IVF)
Stimulating hormones (injectables) are used to stimulate multiple egg production; ultrasounds (scans) monitor response of ovaries to hormones; mature follicles are retrieved (egg retrieval) and fertilized with sperm in the IVF clinic lab (fertilization); resulting day-three embryo or day-five blastocyst is transferred into the uterus (transfer); medication continues and blood test is taken to confirm pregnancy ten days post transfer (pregnancy test).

Fresh Cycle versus Frozen Cycle
A fresh cycle is when embryos or blastocysts are transferred a few days after retrieval from an IVF cycle. Frozen cycles are when embryos or blastocysts have been frozen from a fresh IVF cycle and thawed for transfer.

ICSI—Intracytoplasmic Sperm Injection
It is an IVF-related procedure in which a single sperm is injected directly into an egg to enable fertilization. It is used as treatment for poor sperm motility or morphology.

CCS—Comprehensive Chromosomal Screening, or PGD— Preimplantation Genetic Diagnosis

To reduce potential miscarriage rate and passage of genetic problems to off-spring, CCS (previously called PGD) is an IVF-related procedure in which an embryo biopsy is performed on day five after retrieval to test for genetic abnormalities. For single gene disorders, PGD is used, and embryos are biopsied on day three or day five.

Selective Reduction

It reduces a multiple pregnancy (high risk), typically to twins, prior to completion of the third month of pregnancy through injection of a chemical under ultrasound guidance.

SET—Single Embryo Transfer, or DET—Double Embryo Transfer

SET is typically recommended over DET. SET avoids or minimizes the possibility of twins, which carry an increased rate of miscarriage, premature delivery, or birth problems. On rare occasion, a single embryo splits, resulting in identical twins.

Medication

Clomid—Clomiphene Citrate

An oral synthetic hormone to induce ovulation of more than one egg. Often used to enhance fertility in IUIs and to regulate cycle for PCOS.

Heparin

A drug sometimes used during an IVF cycle to prevent blood clotting within the fluid that harbors the egg.

Metformin

An oral diabetic agent used to treat PCOS. Improves insulin sensitivity.

Third-Party Parenting (When DNA or Gestation Is Provided by a Third Party or Donor)

THE PEOPLE

- *Intended Parent (IP)*. Parents from third-party reproduction (egg, sperm, or embryo donation) or surrogacy.
- *Adoptive Parents and Birth Mothers*. Parents from adoption are adoptive parents. Women who relinquish their children for adoption are birth mothers.
- *Sperm Donor*. Men who donate their sperm to an intended parent(s) for IUI or IVF. Donors are matched (primarily anonymously) through a sperm bank or cryobank. Donors willing to be contacted by the child when eighteen years old or older maintain contact information on the donor registry. Sperm donors are called "proven donors" if pregnancy has been confirmed and "known donors" if they are a family member of the intended parent(s) or a friend (not recommended).
- *Egg Donor*. Women who donate their eggs to an intended parent(s) for donor IVF. Donors are matched (primarily anonymously) through an agency, egg bank, or clinic program. Donors willing to be contacted by the child when eighteen years old or older maintain contact information with the agency or clinic program. Egg donors are called "repeat donors" if they have previously donated and "known donors" if they are a family member of the intended parent(s) or a friend (not recommended).
- *Embryo Donor*. Intended parent(s) who donate their extra frozen embryos once their family is complete to another individual or couple via embryo donor program.
- *Gestational Carrier, or Family Surrogate*. Women who carry the pregnancy for an intended parent(s) unable to carry a pregnancy. Gestational carriers are matched (nonanonymously) through an agency and may be first-time or repeat carriers. Intended parents may

match independently with a family member. Additionally, independent arrangements may be matched via surrogacy websites or on own (both not recommended). Women who become pregnant via IUI with the intended father's sperm or donor sperm are referred to as family surrogates (not recommended).

THE OPTIONS

- *Adoption.* Adoptions are arranged through an agency or attorney. Options include domestic adoption, international adoption, or fost-adopt. Domestic adoptions are open (meet and establish some relationship with the birth mother), while international adoption is often closed (do not meet birth mother).
- *Sperm Donation.* Sperm from a donor (obtained from sperm bank, friend, or family member) via AI, IUI, or IVF.
- *Egg Donation.* Eggs from a donor (obtained from agency, egg bank, or clinic program) via IVF. Most commonly recommended for diminished ovarian reserve (DOR). Under ideal conditions, clinics quote a 60–80 percent success rate (given multiple transfers).
- *Embryo Donation.* Extra frozen embryos from an IVF or donor IVF cycle donated to an embryo donor program (clinic or agency based). Embryos are transferred to the intended parent (similar to IUI procedure).
- *Surrogacy.* Gestational surrogacy is when embryos are transferred to a gestational carrier. Donor gestational surrogacy is when embryos from an intended parent's donor IVF cycle are transferred to a gestational carrier. Traditional surrogacy is when the family surrogate becomes pregnant via IUI with the intended father's sperm or donor sperm (not recommended).

Resources

Mindfulness

BARRE CENTER FOR BUDDHIST STUDIES
bcbsdharma.org

BUDDHIST INFORMATION AND EDUCATION NETWORK
buddhanet.net

CENTER FOR MINDFULNESS—UNIVERSITY OF MASSACHUSETTS MEDICAL SCHOOL (JON KABAT-ZINN; SAKI SANTORELLI)
umassmed.edu/cfm

CENTER FOR MINDFULNESS AT UC SAN DIEGO HEALTH
health.ucsd.edu/specialties/mindfulness

PEMA CHODRON
shambhala.org/teachers/pema-chodron
gampoabbey.org

COMPASSION CULTIVATION TRAINING
ccare.stanford.edu

DAILY DHARMA
tricycle.org

STEVE FLOWERS
mindfullivingprograms.com

CHRISTOPHER GERMER
mindfulselfcompassion.org

THICH NHAT HANH
plumvillage.org

INSIGHT MEDITATION CENTERS—WORLD WIDE
buddhanet.net/wbd

INSIGHT MEDITATION CENTER—REDWOOD CITY, CA (GIL FRONSDAL; ANDREA FELLA)
insightmeditationcenter.org

INSIGHT MEDITATION SOUTH BAY—MOUNTAIN VIEW, CA (SHAILA CATHERINE)
imsb.org

INSIGHT MEDITATION SOCIETY, BARRE, MA (JOSEPH GOLDSTEIN; SHARON SALZBERG; AND OTHERS)
dharma.org

JANETTI MAROTTA
janettimarotta.com

KRISTIN NEFF
self-compassion.org

SKILLFUL MEANS (PRACTICES WITH SPIRITUAL AND PSYCHOLOGICAL EMPHASIS)
yourskillfulmeans.com

SPIRIT ROCK (JACK KORNFIELD; SYLVIA BOORSTEIN; AND OTHERS)
spiritrock.com

BOB STAHL
mindfulnessprograms.com

Infertility

AMERICAN PREGNANCY ASSOCIATION
americanpregnancy.org

AMERICAN SOCIETY FOR REPRODUCTIVE MEDICINE (ASRM)
asrm.org

ADOPTION GUIDE
adoptionguide.com

ARC FERTILITY (ADVANCED REPRODUCTIVE CARE, INC.) (NETWORK OF FERTILITY SPECIALISTS, SUPPORT SERVICES, AND FINANCING PROGRAMS)
arcfertility.com

BLUE OVA HEALTH & ACUPUNCTURE (ROBIN SHEARED, LAC)
blueova.com

CREATING A FAMILY: THE NATIONAL INFERTILITY & ADOPTION EDUCATION NONPROFIT
creatingafamily.org

DONOR CONCEPTION NETWORK (SERIES OF BOOKS ON DISCLOSURE DOWNLOADED FREE)
donor-conception-network.org/telltalkpubs.htm

FERTILITY RESOURCES
ihr.com

INFERTILITY NETWORK
infertilitynetworkuk.com

MENTAL-HEALTH SCREENING TOOLS
mentalhealthamerica.net

NATIONAL COUNCIL FOR ADOPTION: ADOPTION ADVOCACY AND AWARENESS
adoptioncouncil.org

ORGANIZATION OF PARENTS THROUGH SURROGACY (OPTS)
opts.com

PALO ALTO MEDICAL FOUNDATION (PAMF) FERTILITY PHYSICIANS
pamf.org/fertility

RESOLVE: THE NATIONAL INFERTILITY ORGANIZATION
resolve.org

SANDS (MISCARRIAGE, STILLBIRTH OR NEONATAL DEATH)
sands.org.au www.sandsforum.org

References

Akhter, S., M. Marcus, R. A. Kerber, M. Kong, and K. C. Taylor. 2016. "The Impact of Periconceptional Maternal Stress on Fecundability." *Annals of Epidemiology* 26 (10): 710–16.e7. https://doi.org/10.1016/j.annepidem.2016.07.015.

Boivin, J., and S. Gameiro. 2015. "Evolution of Psychology and Counseling in Infertility." *Fertility and Sterility* 104 (2): 251–59.

Boivin, J., L. Scanlan, and S. Walker. 1999. "Why Are Infertile Patients not Using Psychosocial Counseling?" *Human Reproduction* 14:1384–91.

Brach, T. 2012. *True Refuge: Finding Peace and Freedom in Your Own Awakened Heart.* New York: Random House.

Burns, D. 1980. *Feeling Good: The New Mood Therapy.* New York: Harper Collins Publishers.

Burns, D. 1990. *The Feeling Good Handbook.* New York: Penguin Books.

Campagne, D. 2006. "Should Fertilization Treatment Start with Reducing Stress?" *Human Reproduction* 21:1651–58.

Catherine, S. 2008. *Focused and Fearless: A Meditator's Guide to States of Deep Joy, Calm, and Clarity.* Somerville, MA: Wisdom Publications.

Chavarro, J., W. Willett, and P. Skerrett. 2008. *The Fertility Diet: Groundbreaking Research Reveals Natural Ways to Boost Ovulation and Improve Your Chances of Getting Pregnant*. New York: McGraw Hill Companies.

Chen, T. H., S. P. Chang, C. F. Tsai, and K. D. Juang. 2004. "Prevalence of Depressive and Anxiety Disorders in an Assisted Reproductive Technique Clinic." *Human Reproduction* 19 (10): 2313–18.

Chodron, P. 2000. *When Things Fall Apart: Heart Advice for Difficult Times*. Boston: Shambhala.

Cooper-Hilbert, B. 1998. *Infertility and Involuntary Childlessness: Helping Couples Cope*. New York: W. W. Norton & Company.

Daniels, K. 2004. *Building a Family with the Assistance of Donor Insemination*. Palmerston North, New Zealand: Dunmore Press.

Davidson, R. J., J. Kabat-Zinn, J. Schumacher, M. Rosenkranz, D. Muller, S. F. Santorelli, F. Urbanowski, A. Harrington, K. Bonus, and J. F. Sheridan. 2003. "Alterations in Brain and Immune Function Produced by Mindfulness Meditation." *Psychosomatic Medicine* 65:564–70.

Deveraux, L., and A. J. Hammerman. 1998. *Infertility & Identity*. San Francisco: Jossey-Bass Publishers.

Domar, A. 2004. "Impact of Psychological Factors on Dropout Rates in Insured Infertility Patients." *Fertility and Sterility* 81:271–73.

Domar, A. 2015. "Creating a Collaborative Model of Mental Health Counseling for the Future." *Fertility and Sterility* 104 (2): 277–80.

Domar, A. D., K. Smith, L. Conboy, M. Iannone, and M. Alper. 2010. "A Prospective Investigation into the Reasons Why Insured United States

Patients Drop Out of In Vitro Fertilization Treatment." *Fertility and Sterility* 94:1457–59.

Domar, A. D., P. C. Zuttermeister, and R. Friedman. 1993. "The Psychological Impact of Infertility: A Comparison to Patients with Other Medical Conditions." *Journal of Psychosomatic Obstetrics & Gynecology* 14:45–52.

Ehrensaft, D. 2005. *Mommies, Daddies, Donors, Surrogates: Answering Tough Questions and Building Strong Families.* New York: Guilford Press.

Emmons, R. 2007. *Thanks! How the New Science of Gratitude Can Make You Happier.* New York: Houghton Mifflin.

Eugster, A. and A. L. Vingerhoets. 1999. "Psychological Aspects of In Vitro Fertilization: A Review." *Social Science & Medicine* 48 (5): 575–89.

Frederiksen, Y., I. Farver-Vestergaard, N. G. Skovgard, H. J. Ingerslev, and R. Zachariae. 2015. "Efficacy of Psychosocial Interventions for Psychological and Pregnancy Outcomes in Infertile Women and Men: A Systematic Review and Meta-Analysis." *BMJ Open* 5: e006592.

Freeman, E. W., A. S. Boxer, K. Rickels, R. Tureck, and L. Mastrionni. 1985. "Psychological Evaluation and Support in a Program of In Vitro Fertilization and Embryo Transfer." *Fertility and Sterility* 43:48–53.

Fronsdal, G. 2001. *The Issue at Hand: Essays on Buddhist Mindfulness Practice.* Redwood City, CA: Insight Meditation Center.

Gameiro, S., J. Boivin, and C. M. Verhaak. 2012. "Why Do Patients Discontinue Fertility Treatment? A Systematic Review of Reasons and Predictors of Discontinuation in Fertility Treatment." *Human Reproduction Update* 18 (6): 652–69.

Germer, C., R. Siegel, and P. Fulton. 2005. *Mindfulness and Psychotherapy.* New York: Guilford Press.

Goldin, P. 2010. "Effect of Mindfulness Training on the Neural Bases of Emotion Regulation in Social Anxiety Disorder." Paper presented at the Center for Mindfulness Conference, Worchester, MA.

Gray, J. 1992. *Men Are from Mars, Women Are from Venus: A Practical Guide for Improving Communication & Getting What You Want in Your Relationships.* New York: Harper Collins.

Greenfeld, D. 2015. "Effects and Outcomes of Third-Party Reproduction: Parents." *Fertility and Sterility* 104 (3): 520–24.

Hanson, R. 2009. *Buddha's Brain: The Practical Neuroscience of Happiness, Love, and Wisdom.* Oakland, CA: New Harbinger Publications.

Hayes, S. 2005. *Get Out of Your Mind and into Your Life: The New Acceptance and Commitment Therapy.* Oakland, CA: New Harbinger Publications.

Hullender Rubin, L., M. Opsahl, K. Wiemer, S. Mist, and A. Caughey. 2015. "Impact of Whole Systems Traditional Chinese Medicine on In Vitro Fertilization Outcomes." *Reproductive BioMedicine Online* 30 (6): 602–12.

Kabat-Zinn, J. 1990. *Full Catastrophe Living: Using the Wisdom of Your Body and Mind to Face Stress, Pain, and Illness.* New York: Dell.

Kabat-Zinn, J. 2005. *Coming to Our Senses: Healing Ourselves and the World through Mindfulness.* New York: Hyperion.

Kabat-Zinn, J. 2013. *Full Catastrophe Living (Revised Edition): Using the Wisdom of Your Body and Mind to Face Stress, Pain, and Illness.* New York: Bantam Books.

Kornfield, J. 2008. *The Wise Heart: A Guide to the Universal Teachings of Buddhist Psychology.* New York: Bantam Books.

Kubler-Ross, E. 1969. *On Death and Dying: What the Dying Have to Teach Doctors, Nurses, Clergy and Their Own Families.* New York: Simon & Schuster.

Kung, C. 2006. *Heart of a Buddha.* Taiwan: Amitabha Publications.

Levine, S. 1979. *A Gradual Awakening.* New York: Anchor Books.

Lutz, A., J. Brefczynski-Lewis, T. Johnstone, and R. J. Davidson. 2008a. "Regulation of the Neural Circuitry of Emotion by Compassion Meditation: Effects of Meditative Expertise." *PLOS One* 3 (3): e1897.

Lutz, A., H. A. Slagter, J. D. Dunne, and R. J. Davidson. 2008b. "Attention Regulation and Monitoring in Meditation." *Trends in Cognitive Sciences* 12 (4): 163–69.

Marotta, J. 2013. *50 Mindful Steps to Self-Esteem: Everyday Practices for Cultivating Self-Acceptance and Self-Compassion.* Oakland, CA: New Harbinger Publications.

Moffitt, P. 2002. "Selfless Gratitude." *Yoga Journal* 168:61–66.

Neff, K. 2011. *Self-Compassion: Stop Beating Yourself Up and Leave Insecurity Behind.* New York: Harper Collins.

Nhat Hanh, T. 1976. *The Miracle of Mindfulness: An Introduction to the Practice of Meditation.* Boston: Beacon Press.

Nhat Hanh, T. 1992. *Peace Is Every Step. The Path of Mindfulness in Everyday Life.* New York: Bantam Books.

Nhat Hanh, T. 2004. *Mindful Living.* Boulder, CO: Sounds True.

Paulus, W., M. Zhang, E. Strehler, I. El-Danasouri, and K. Sterzil. 2002. "Influence of Acupuncture on the Pregnancy Rate in Patients Who Undergo Assisted Reproduction Therapy." *Fertility and Sterility* 77:721–24.

Pei, J., E. Strehler, U. Noss, A. Markus, P. Piomboni, B. Baccetti, and K. Sterzik. 2005. "Quantitative Evaluation of Spermatozoa Ultrastructure after Acupuncture Treatment for Idiopathic Male Infertility." *Fertility and Sterility* 84 (1): 141–47.

Ryan, M. J. 2007. *Giving Thanks: The Gifts of Gratitude.* San Francisco: Conari Press.

Ryan, M. J. 2009. *Attitudes of Gratitude.* San Francisco: Red Wheel/Weiser.

Salzberg, S. 2002. *Lovingkindness: The Revolutionary Art of Happiness.* Boston: Shambhala.

Sandberg, S. and A. Grant. 2017. *Option B: Finding Adversity, Building Resilience, and Finding Joy.* New York: Knopf.

Schlaff, W. and A. Braverman. 2015. "Introduction: Role of Mental Health Professionals in the Care of Infertile Patients." *Fertility and Sterility* 104 (2): 249–50.

Siegel, B. 1986. *Love, Medicine and Miracles: Lessons Learned about Self-Healing from a Surgeon's Experience with Exceptional Patients.* New York: Harper & Row, Publishers.

Siegel, D. 2010. *Mindsight: The New Science of Personal Transformation.* New York: Bantam Books.

Smeenk, J., C. Verhaak, A. Stolwijk, J. Kremer, and D. Braat. 2004. "Reasons for Dropout in an In Vitro Fertilization/Intracytophasmic Sperm Injection Program." *Fertility and Sterility* 77:505–10.

Speroff L., R. H. Glass, and N. G. Kase. 1999. *Clinical Gynecologic Endocrinology and Infertility 6th Edition*. Baltimore, MD: Lippincott Williams and Wilkens.

Stahl, B. and E. Goldstein. 2010. *Mindfulness-Based Stress Reduction Workbook*. Oakland, CA: New Harbinger Publications.

Weil, A. 2005. *Dr. Andrew Weil's Mindbody Tool Kit*. Boulder, CO: Sounds True.

Young, S. 2004. *Break through Pain: A Step-by-Step Mindfulness Program for Transforming Chronic and Acute Pain*. Boulder, CO: Sounds True.

Zweifel, J. 2015. "Donor Conception from the Viewpoint of the Child: Positives, Negative, and Promoting the Welfare of the Child." *Fertility and Sterility* 104 (3): 513–19.

About the Author

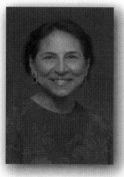

Janetti Marotta, PhD, shares the lessons of her own healing journey through infertility, and those of the women and men she has worked with, to bring the teaching and practice of mindfulness to the challenge of fertility. After five years of repeated miscarriages, IVFs, donor IVFs, and failed adoptions, she became the mother of a daughter through surrogacy. She is a clinical psychologist, published author, featured speaker, and workshop facilitator and has specialized in every area of infertility since 1990.

Dr. Marotta is a graduate of Yale University and the University of Nevada, Reno, who has served on the regional board of RESOLVE, the National Infertility Organization, and worked as a staff psychologist in the Department of Psychiatry at Stanford University. She is the founder of the Fertility Support and Mindfulness Program at Palo Alto Medical Foundation Fertility Physicians. Dr. Marotta is a long-time practitioner of meditation and mindfulness and also author of the book *50 Mindful Steps to Self-Esteem: Everyday Practices for Cultivating Self-Acceptance and Self-Compassion*. For more information about her work, you may visit her website, www.janettimarotta.com.

Accessories to A Fertile Path!

Free ten-minute guided meditations that complement each chapter's formal practice are available on www.janettimarotta.com/meditations.

Made in the USA
Monee, IL
09 November 2019